T0367885

ENDORSEMENT

"Mary is a living testimony to God's healing grace, and, through the Holy Spirit's guidance, has recovered God's hidden secrets concerning health and long life."

—Dr. Barbie Breathitt, Breath of the Spirit Ministries, www.MyOnar.com

CANCER
How I Beat It on a Shoestring Budget!

YOU DON'T
HAVE TO BE
CANCER'S
NEXT
VICTIM

MARY ROCK

WESTBOW°
PRESS
A DIVISION OF THOMAS NELSON
& ZONDERVAN

WestBow Press books may be ordered through booksellers or by contacting:

WestBow Press
A Division of Thomas Nelson & Zondervan
1663 Liberty Drive
Bloomington, IN 47403
www.westbowpress.com
1 (866) 928-1240

ISBN: 978-1-4908-7371-8 (sc)
ISBN: 978-1-4908-7372-5 (e)

Library of Congress Control Number: 2015904859

Print information available on the last page.

WestBow Press rev. date: 10/5/2015

To my wonderful mother, Lucy Ashmore Fagan, who succumbed to the disease of ovarian cancer on December 17, 1999. Mama, your heartfelt and powerful prayer paved the way for the saving of many lives.

With very special thanks to my husband, Daniel Patrick Rock, a man who loves God and never stopped encouraging me to write.

A special thank you to Melissa Krueger of Lakeland, Florida, who lent her expertise in the use of essential oils.

Contents

Foreword

I met Mary and Dan Rock several years ago during their attendance at one of our Sunday morning meetings at The Covenant Center in Lakeland, Florida. Although they lived over an hour away, Mary and Dan began to attend and participate regularly. In time Mary privately shared with my wife the miraculous testimony of her swift healing and recovery of Stage 4 breast cancer by following instructions she received in a dream, which guided her toward a natural approach to healing.

I have found Mary and Dan to be genuinely caring, compassionate and generous individuals who truly hunger for the presence of God. Mary has the heart of a worshipper and delights in expressing to others the joy and humor of God found in daily living.

A common thread, in the many prophetic words spoken over Mary, has been for her to write. This book is a result of her obedience and desire to share her healing journey and testimony, including various natural alternative methods that may assist and promote the healing process.

Over the years Mary has exhibited relentless faith through her life challenges, including her husband suffering a health crisis that nearly took his life. She is a woman of prayer, peace, and perseverance who has witnessed God's faithfulness and diversity of healing and miracles. I have observed Holy Spirit strengthening Mary through each hardship and have found her to be stalwart and relentless in her attacking each challenge with faith and determination.

Mary Rock has something significant to say not only to the body of Christ, but the entire world. This informative book clearly outlines and presents to the reader for consideration, an affordable natural alternative approach to gaining victory over cancer. The testimonials of individuals who have successfully followed this same natural approach will bring hope and encouragement to those who now search for the door to their physical healing.

Richard Maisenbacher, Pastor
The Covenant Center

Preface

Dear Reader,

I first must say that anything I have written in this book is not medical advice, but rather educational information that I have gathered. It is against the law for anyone without a physician's license to offer medical advice in the USA. I am not a doctor. I have merely written my personal testimony and related the testimonies of others, and I am only able to share what worked for me and for them. This work should not be construed as any kind of attempt to either prescribe or practice medicine.

Most, if not all, of the information contained in this book is available on the Internet, and I have simply restated it here. It is my hope to save you hours of research.

I have been asked by the Lord to share my wonderful story of victory, providing hope to others. This work is the result of His request.

Mary Rock

SECTION 1

Experience: The Very Best Teacher

Quick Start Guide

This book contains easy steps I took to recover from cancer and maintain good health.

To get an overview of how I fought breast cancer refer to Chapter 3. Chapter 3 includes the method for the castor oil pack I used on the tumor and the specific protocol I used that is geared toward breast cancer and other lymphatic cancers.

Chapter 18 and Chapter 19 contain the instructions I followed in my successful encounter with ovarian cancer and learned this approach would be appropriate for all cancers; I learned the detox trio and herbal germ cleanse can be taken by anyone who is interested in maintaining a healthy lifestyle and creating an environment in the body that is hostile to the growth of cancer.

Chapter 21 explains what I learned about the importance of bowel cleansing while battling any cancer, and in Chapter 22, I share my experience with an amazingly effective product I used for just pennies a day.

In Chapter 36, you will find a list of supplements I found useful.

CHAPTER 1

My Answer Was in the Garden

*With the ancient is wisdom; and in length of
days understanding. —Job 12:12 KJV*

Long before Adam and Eve sinned in the Garden of Eden, an act which opened the door of disease unto all creation, God in His wisdom anticipated their failure and provided the herbal remedies necessary to recover from all sickness, including the disease of cancer.

The following account is the wisdom that God—in His mercy, kindness, and grace—granted me, bringing rapid restoration to my health. I now joyfully share this wonderful, life-saving information.

There are many books written about the natural cure for cancer. Most of those books require tremendous human effort and a drastic change of lifestyle, promising positive results when there is strict adherence to the recommended program, as well as a timely undertaking of the prescribed approach.

This book is different in that I reveal a form of medicine practiced for thousands of years by ancient peoples who were well aware of the bounty God had provided in the Garden. These ancient peoples knew how to use herbal remedies to stop the growth of a tumor. They realized these herbal remedies could also dismantle the tumor.

Regardless of where a person may be in their battle with cancer, this revelation of an ancient practice of medicine brings renewed hope.

Many may find this difficult to believe, yet a turnaround in my health took place in just a few hours. A physician may say it's too late and to get your affairs in order. Conversely, God's infallible word tells us the leaves of the trees are for the healing of the nations. I chose to believe God's word and here I am healed and proclaiming it is not too late, and it is not impossible!

In my case of stage 4 breast cancer, within just a few hours of taking the herbal remedy, the malignancy retreated. The normal color began to quickly return to the once swollen, crimson, throbbing breast and the baseball-sized tumor rapidly began to shrink. The tumor was quickly dismantled by the proper herbal supplements, detoxification and simple lifestyle changes.

I share in this book the easy steps I followed to recover from cancer. I list the inexpensive yet powerful herbal products I used, which were easily obtained and proved to be completely effective in ridding my body of malignancy. Additionally, I share what foods I learned to avoid and what foods helped bring about healing in my body.

I also disclose an inexpensive product I now take which aids me in maintaining my good health, costing me just pennies a day.

I have written a chapter filled solely with the amazing testimonies of others who crossed my path and were healed of end stage cancers when they followed the same simple steps; one of these individuals had been informed by his physician he had only 3 weeks to live!

I invite the reader to follow my journey as I relate what I discovered: the simple reasons cancer has become such a rampant disease and the easy steps to take to avoid becoming cancer's next victim.

The curtain is pulled back and the secret is revealed.

CHAPTER 2

It Began with a Dream from God

I the Lord will make myself known unto him in a vision,
and will speak unto him in a dream.—Numbers 12:6 KJV

The week prior to having the dream I will share with you, I spent several days praying for hours at a time. Rather than the usual things I often find myself in prayer about—protection, provision, prayer requests from others—I felt myself drawn by the Holy Spirit into a wonderful time of almost effortless prayer. There was no critical situation I was aware of which pressed me into prayer. If I were to ever experience this glorious phenomenon again, I would realize immediately there was something on the horizon I was not equipped to handle successfully without God's supernatural intervention.

I had attended a monthly women's meeting at my church Saturday morning and was exhausted by the time I arrived home in the afternoon. I told my husband I was going to lie down and rest. I fell fast asleep and began to dream.

I dreamed two little girls and I were taken captive by two evil, men-like creatures, which looked like gargoyles, those grotesque creatures that serve as waterspouts on the corners of many old buildings. The little girls and I were trapped in the back seat of an old truck one of the men was driving. I had no idea who these little girls were, but I felt an overwhelming sense of responsibility to protect them. The two men holding us captive were each armed with sawed-off shotguns they brandished about recklessly, and they threatened repeatedly to kill the little girls and me.

7

The old, beat-up truck we were all in zoomed down the road at an extremely high rate of speed. Suddenly, the truck crashed full-speed into a white wall, which turned out to be the outside wall of a store. I seized the opportunity to leap from the truck and said to the two men that I would go around the corner and get something for them. They were unable to stop me or follow me, but stayed in their vehicle with the little girls.

I knew that the little girls were being held as hostages and in very great danger—that they were powerless to do anything for themselves. I knew I alone had the responsibility of getting help, or they were going to die at the hands of these two evil men.

I ran around the corner and opened the door of the store. As soon as I entered the store, I began to shout to the store employees to lock the door and call 911. The store employees did exactly what I asked of them, but their reaction to my predicament was so calm and detached from my state of panic, that I was even more unnerved. The fact that those evil men were holding the little girls captive outside the store had me panic-stricken.

The employee who was behind the counter had very large eyes, and the other store employee, a young man named Michael, walked around as if he did not have a care in the world. Because of what I perceived as a completely nonchalant attitude in a very dire crisis, I ran up an available staircase, found a red telephone at the top of the stairs and called 911 for myself.

When I made contact with the police dispatch person, she told me I needed to calm down—that I should look out the window from the second story and see the police were already on the scene and had everything fully under control. I pulled back the curtain in front of the window, looked down from the second story, and saw the police had completely surrounded the truck, taken the two evil men into custody, and slapped a pair of handcuffs on the one man who was sitting on the left-hand side of the truck. The little girls were safe and sound!

When I awoke from this dream, I had no inkling as to what it meant. I only knew it was alarming, but, most importantly, the dream had a desirable and peaceful outcome. At that very moment, I lifted my hands toward heaven and began thanking God for giving me an answer of peace.

A few weeks before I had the dream, my husband and I were at our church on a Thursday night. Our pastor called the entire congregation up for prayer. When I was prayed for, the pastor mentioned the Holy Spirit had said to pray for my chest. I gave some thought as to why the Holy Spirit instructed the pastor to pray over my chest, but I did not have any fear about it at all and soon forgot about it altogether.

Ordinarily, I would have mulled this over in my mind endlessly in an effort to come to some kind of resolution as to what God was saying, but not this time. I had perfect peace about it.

Several days passed, and I awoke on a Monday morning with a slight ache in my left breast. I totally dismissed it. It wasn't too painful, so I was easily able to ignore it. I was so focused on accomplishing the tasks at hand that I didn't give it a second thought.

My husband, Daniel, a busy attorney, was involved in a weeklong trial in the county of Hillsborough, and the Hillsborough County Courthouse was nearly an hour's drive away. It was my job to make sure he looked good for the courtroom.

I was busy running errands, shopping, going to the dry cleaners, and steaming wrinkles out of his ties and sweater vests, as we were experiencing some unusually cold weather.

I juiced fresh vegetables for him every morning that week to give him extra energy and packed him additional fresh juice and snacks to go, because his days were so long and arduous, leaving him little or no time for a healthy lunch. He was working on the case constantly, even during Court recesses. He did not return home from Court in Tampa until very late each evening, and even then he was up until the wee hours of each night, doing research and preparing for the next day of trial.

So there was a lot of energy flowing through the house, and I was focused on doing my part and very aware of the fact my husband did not need any distractions. His focus needed to be on the trial. When it comes to his clients, his attitude is always winning is everything! He is an extremely competitive and focused person with a fine reputation among his peers as an unrelenting and aggressive opponent in Court. I was determined not to get in his way, but to do everything I could that week to help him.

Another day passed at the Rock household, though, and the situation with my breast had worsened. My left breast began throbbing, was now swollen, and somewhat discolored with a bruised appearance, red and

9

slightly purplish. I did not feel well and experienced unquenchable thirst. I also had no appetite. I felt concerned but pressed on with everything I needed to do that day, thinking I would discuss the matter with my husband at the end of his busy week.

However, by the following morning, my breast was even worse. In addition to the constant throbbing, nearly my entire left breast had turned crimson, with a bruised appearance. My breast had become somewhat transparent, exposing strange-looking, evenly spaced linear streaks of white beneath my skin, and my breast was now much more swollen. The veins in my breast were also very prominent, and I finally realized this was extremely serious. This was not a small lump which could be detected through diagnostic testing; this was now a swollen, throbbing, full-blown mass the size of a baseball.

For two nights in a row, I had taken ibuprofen because the constant throbbing in my breast prevented me from falling asleep. I felt hot, feverish and dehydrated, drinking nearly a gallon of water during the night trying to quench my thirst.

Recognizing the fact this was not going to keep until the end of the week, I showed my breast to my husband. He was extremely alarmed, and as he left for Court early that morning, he gave me strict instructions to contact my doctor immediately. Incredibly, I still did not have a full grasp on the severity of the situation, even though a large, throbbing mass the size of a baseball was bulging from my left breast. Obviously, I was experiencing some denial. Mercifully, my husband did not say what was on his mind, and this helped prevent me from going into a total panic. Instead this allowed me to remain in peace as a very menacing situation gradually unfolded.

I called my OB/GYN's office promptly at nine that morning, hoping he could see me that day, describing my symptoms and the appearance of my breast to the nurse. To my surprise, the nurse did not even want me to come in to the office but instead gave me the name and number of another doctor and said I should call her office immediately. I naively asked the nurse what the doctor's specialty was, and with just a hint of exasperation in her voice, she replied that the doctor was a surgeon at a well-known cancer treatment center in Tampa. I overheard a distant whispered voice on the other end of the phone, saying, "Oh, no, not another one." When I hung up the phone, I was stunned.

I quickly went to my computer and typed in the phrase "photos of stage 4 breast cancers." My breast appeared identical to several of the photos, and in some cases, my breast looked even worse than the photos that came up during the search. My first thought was that everyone I knew who had been treated at this cancer treatment center was either missing a body part or now dead. I quickly dismissed the nurse's recommendation to call the surgeon.

Incredibly, I still thought I had options! I had a tremendous amount of peace all about me—not even an inkling of panic—yet I was acutely aware I had to seek out a solution. I realized I certainly could not just ignore what was going on, but I was not at all frightened. Now, believe me, this had to be the supernatural peace of God. This reaction alone is a testimony to the power of prayer. Through prayer, God had given me the insight into making a decision based on His infallible wisdom, rather than choosing the fallible knowledge of conventional medicine.

Even though my own mother died of ovarian cancer, I had never really allowed myself to seriously ponder what actions I would take if I developed the disease of cancer. I never permitted my mind to go there. In my mind, cancer was a disease which happened to other people. Up to that point, if someone had found they were suffering with a throbbing breast tumor the size of a baseball, the obvious solution to me would have been to seek the help of a physician. Yet suddenly, seeing a physician did not seem like the right thing for me to do.

I immediately called Hannah, the lady who manages a local health food store and gave her a quick explanation. Hannah lives near my home and would stop by my house two or three times a week to drop off organic groceries and other natural products I ordered from her over the phone. She told me she would be at my house in exactly one hour.

Later, after I had the time to sit back, take in the entire experience, and reflect on my dream in depth, I realized the wall of the store the old truck hit was the health food store. The person behind the counter with the big eyes represented Hannah and the wisdom she possessed. The person, Michael (a name which means "Who is like God?"), who was walking about so peacefully and nonchalantly, represented the ease with which I would achieve a healing for breast cancer.

The curtains, which I pulled back, meant that by my own hand, I would reveal what had previously been hidden from many—namely, the easy solution for recovering from cancer. I also realized a much deeper meaning of the wall the truck hit was that it was the Lord. "For I, says the Lord, will be unto her a wall" (Zechariah 2:5 KJV).

Hannah arrived in an hour, just as she promised. By that time, the severity of the situation had really begun to sink in. The throbbing in my breast had become so intense I had applied an icepack in an effort to get some relief. Hannah was fully confident I would be okay, and she gave me the same soothing and reassuring response each of the two or three times when I asked—now with some genuine concern—whether this was going to work.

Hannah pulled five products out of the bag that added up to less than $50 and gave me some quick instructions and left to go back to her job at the store.

While I carried out her instructions, the meaning of the dream I'd had only days before with regard to the little girls flooded my mind, and I was immediately filled with confidence. It finally dawned on me "the little girls" were my breasts, and I suddenly realized the two grotesque men-like creatures in the dream, who were threatening to kill the little girls and me, were cancer and death. They were stopped when their truck hit the wall and they were subsequently arrested and taken into custody. In my dream, I saw the creature who was sitting on the left side of the truck arrested and handcuffed, and the tumor was in my left breast.

A number of other dreams I'd had recently also began to make sense. They were warnings from God about the danger of the bio-identical estrogen cream I had been applying. In an attempt to stop the hot flashes I had experienced for the past several months, I had applied the cream too liberally. The estrogen cream had caused the rapid growth of the tumor. I had been warned many times by my physician and by my pharmacist about the dangers of estrogen cream, but I chose to ignore the warnings, instead focusing only on some way to get relief from the awful menopausal symptoms I experienced at the time.

The results of applying estrogen cream or swallowing an estrogen capsule, any estrogenic product, manmade or natural, when a breast tumor is present is somewhat akin to pouring gasoline on a fire; the result will be an explosion of growth—exactly what I experienced. I subsequently discovered that as a result of suffering with a hormonal cancer, I also had to avoid progesterone and testosterone supplementation.

My husband arrived home several hours later that day, and as soon as he set his foot inside the door, he promptly set about questioning me as to whether I had called the doctor. When I responded that the lady from the health food store had brought me something to take care of the problem, my great big, handsome, and very practical husband in the sharp-looking suit began to raise his voice at me in frustration, telling me in a very heated tone—actually, it ever so slightly resembled yelling at me, but he asked me not to say that—I had given myself breast cancer with the hormones I had been using, and I needed to go to the hospital for treatment immediately.

Completely out of character for me, I wasn't even rattled by his ominous-sounding words or stern manner. I just very calmly repeated to him the dream I had several days before and continued stirring the homemade soup I was preparing for dinner. He trailed off to our home office to use the computer, most likely too exhausted from arguing all day in Court to try reasoning with me, quickly realizing he wasn't going to win this round.

Typically, if my husband speaks any words of disapproval to me, I go into panic mode while I busily try to think how I can defend my stance. This reaction is shortly followed by a barrage of words from me that don't usually hold much weight with him. Having a dispute with someone who is trained and practiced in the skill of argument can be exasperating.

Later, when my husband was calm and distracted by the task of answering his e-mails, I casually strolled into our home office, as opposed to barging in there, ready to give him a piece of my mind. I gently asked him to give me the definition of the word "arrested." After all, I thought, he's an attorney; the meaning should be obvious to him.

His quick response to me was that it meant "to stop." My response to him was a lightning-quick recitation—he is not too good at listening to my long, drawn-out explanations— of the dream from several days ago. I then gave him a brief interpretation of what I thought the dream actually meant. He didn't say anything else about it that night. He was too busy and too exhausted.

Afterward, I realized God had given my husband supernatural peace because his normal reaction would have been to pick me up, put me in the car, and drive me to the emergency room. I was also aware that God had given me supernatural peace, as well, because ordinarily my first reaction to this type of crisis would have been to panic. I had a great sense of peace about me and no fear whatsoever. I could feel the tangible presence of God's Holy Spirit. I had the sensation, as I walked about my home, of being completely enveloped by His Spirit.

That night, on the very same day Hannah brought me the small bag of items from the health food store, before I retired for the evening, the throbbing in my left breast which I had experienced for more than two days completely stopped! I had improved so dramatically from the time of Hannah's arrival that day that I knew without a doubt I would make a complete recovery.

Early the next morning, my husband informed me he awakened at about 3:00 a.m. from a very strange dream. He dreamed he had gone to a house that was similar to the one I inherited from my parents. He was in the living room of the house and saw a reddish-brown carpet—the color of my hair. The living room in the house was full of dead scorpions; they were all lying on their backs. He realized during his dream the scorpions had eaten something in the house that killed every last one of them.

After he shared his dream with me, we both realized the house in my husband's dream symbolized my body, and the scorpions were the malignant cancer cells. We rejoiced and felt a sense of awe. We realized God had shown me such incredible kindness and mercy. I felt so well the following morning I got dressed and went shopping!

I followed Hannah's instructions to the letter, and the baseball-sized tumor I suffered with shrank within 3 weeks to less than the size of a very small grain of rice. That was where it stopped shrinking. It was tiny, but I knew it was there.

The emergency was over, and I was no longer in danger of losing my breast or dying, but at the time I lacked the information necessary to complete my healing. In Chapter 22, I disclose the inexpensive product I used to recover completely.

As my healing journey progressed, I learned of many pieces of detoxification equipment. I found one of the secrets to staying free of disease is by making a habit of detoxification. I provide a detailed description of these items in Chapter 45. This equipment and many other wonderful natural products that I used to get well and stay well are available on my website, www.ibeatcancers.com.

As I complete this book, six years after first realizing I had breast cancer, I am still absolutely in awe of the speed of my recovery and the speed of recovery experienced by others who chose to use the same path I followed.

CHAPTER 3

How I Beat Breast Cancer

Arise, O Lord, save me, O my God, for thou has
smitten all mine enemies upon the cheek bone;
thou has broken their teeth.—Psalm 3:7

I am not a physician, and I am unqualified to give medical advice in any way. This is an account of how I beat breast cancer.

I learned that I would get the best results by beginning my treatment with the detox trio outlined in Chapter 18, as the detox trio freed up my white blood cells so they could fight the cancer. The following is what worked for me:

1. Juice of Wild Oreganol from North American Herb & Spice Company—three full tablespoons, three times a day; I mixed it with low sodium V-8 juice. This product, as well as the other products listed in this chapter is available on my website, www.ibeatcancers.com.
2. Lymph Cleanse capsules by Solaray—two capsules three times a day.
3. Curcumin capsules (also known as turmeric)—two capsules three times a day. I learned Curcumin is an excellent antifungal and anti-inflammatory that boosts the immune system and shuts off the blood supply to the tumor. NOTE: I learned I should avoid taking Curcumin if I suffered with gallstones.

4. A large bottle of cold pressed castor oil –which I used in a castor oil pack, as well as using it to rebuild my body's immune system, as outlined in Chapter 10.

5. A bag of flax seed, ground in a coffee grinder and eaten—one teaspoon with each meal; I took this by either mixing it in a glass of water or sprinkling it on my food.

I purchased these last four items later. If my budget was tight, just buying the first 5 items listed above would be enough for me to get great results.

6. Zymaclenz capsules—one capsule three times a day. I learned enzymes dismantle or break down a tumor, actually consuming it.

7. Rubinol—a tincture of wild black raspberries; I took a couple of droppers full under the tongue, four times a day. I read that this tincture helps downgrade an aggressive type of breast cancer to a slower growing one, making it a cancer that is weaker and easier to defeat. Dr. Mehmet Oz has mentioned the effectiveness of wild black raspberries as a natural remedy to breast cancer.

8. Purely E— I took five drops three times a day, as I learned that natural source vitamin E softens the hard shell-like cover of the tumor, allowing the other products to more easily penetrate and destroy it. I also learned that eating organic sunflower seeds or organic sunflower seed butter would provide this sort of vitamin E.

9. Chaga tincture or Chaga Black with wild powdered rose hips—I took several drops of the tincture or drank Chaga Black throughout the day, which provides SOD, super oxide dismutase, which rebuilds and strengthens the body, allowing the body's own immune system to fight disease. NOTE: I learned that Chaga should not be consumed while taking antibiotics or chemotherapy.

I learned I could eat seeds, seed butters, nuts, nut butters, lightly steamed vegetables, wild salmon, organic eggs, and fresh organic, free range or wild meats that are slowly and thoroughly cooked. I also learned I could eat meats that are labeled as raised without hormones or antibiotics, preparing them in the same manner, slowly and thoroughly cooked. I learned that adding a tablespoon of apple cider vinegar to the pot, along with a teaspoon of healthy salt when I begin the cooking process will draw important nutrition from the bones. Bone is full of minerals, mostly calcium and phosphorus, along with sodium, magnesium, and other trace minerals that our bodies need to maintain good health.

Hannah recommended that I make a castor oil pack at the tumor site. I saturated a piece of flannel cloth with castor oil, covered the tumor site with the oil-saturated flannel cloth, placed plastic wrap over that, put my bra on to hold it in place, and left it on day and night, removing only when I bathed. I wore a castor oil pack for a couple of weeks straight, changing the pack every day, making sure that it was always well saturated with castor oil. I learned that I could substitute a piece of clean white t-shirt if I didn't have a piece of flannel cloth.

Even though I later learned of other products that were effective in treating cancer in other parts of the body, I learned following this step of applying a castor oil pack to a tumor site would always be appropriate. I read that castor oil is anti-inflammatory, anti-viral, anti-bacterial and antifungal oil, providing the advantage of attacking the tumor externally as well as internally.

I further learned that castor oil also serves to soften the tumor, again allowing the other products to more easily penetrate and dismantle the tumor. Cold pressed castor oil also boosts the immune system. The largest portion of the body's immune system, 70%, is located in the intestines, on the right side of the lower abdomen. I learned the easy and inexpensive steps to strengthen the immune system and shared this information in Chapter 10.

I learned if there had been an open wound because of a cancerous tumor, I would need to wait until the wound had healed before applying a castor oil pack. I learned the Miracle II soaps and Miracle II Neutralizer that I have written about in this book can effectively treat an open cancer wound, as together these products kill bacteria and heal infection. I have written about the wonderful Miracle II products in Chapter 38.

According to what I have read, the Juice of Wild Oreganol and an enzyme product, such as Zymaclenz, along with drinking plenty of medicinal teas will help an open wound heal very quickly.

I also learned that if I was suffering with a bacterial infection, I should take a warm water enema mixed with 2 ounces of Miracle II Neutralizer every day. Chapter 21 explains what I learned about the importance of bowel health.

I later learned that using 35% food grade hydrogen peroxide would aid in cleansing my body of germs, bacteria, cancer and viruses.

I learned what I ate had an impact on whether I would be healed. When I realized I had breast cancer, I was determined to avoid any food that would impede my healing. This meant I immediately stopped eating any grain products, potatoes, fruit, starchy vegetables and dairy products. I learned dairy can inflame certain types of breast cancer, but organic dairy can be very nourishing for those suffering other types of cancer. I also stopped eating sugar, real or artificial, even temporarily eliminating stevia. I learned these foods would feed the cancer and hinder my speedy recovery.

I read an Internet article featuring Travis Christofferson, author of *Tripping Over the Truth: The Metabolic Theory of Cancer.* Christofferson said research has found the ketogenic diet may beat chemotherapy for many forms of cancer. In his book, he quotes a well-known cancer research scientist, Dominic D'Agostino, who said, "Most cancer scientists have historically thought cancer was a genetic disease, but only 5 to 10 percent of cancer is hereditary."

Christofferson learned a low-calorie ketogenic diet combined with oxygen therapy can prevent and significantly reduce the spread of cancer by improving metabolic health. I have written how I very successfully used an inexpensive method of oxygen therapy in Chapter 22.

Researcher D'Agostino told Christofferson that we all have cancerous or pre-cancerous cells growing inside our bodies, but people with healthy immune systems prevent the cancer from becoming established. The mechanisms that keep cells from mutating, the DNA repair process, depend on healthy mitochondrial function. Healthy mitochondria are the ultimate tumor suppressor. D'Agostino says the way to keep mitochondria healthy is through the low-carbohydrate, high fat ketogenic diet, which stimulates mitochondrial biogenesis and enhances mitochondrial efficiency. Christofferson has written what so many in the alternative health field have been saying for years: Cancer cells love carbohydrates. A ketogenic diet starves cancer.

According to Christofferson's research, "The ketogenic diet inhibits the growth of cancer cells by reducing the blood sugar spikes that fuel inflammation." He writes that D'Agostino said, "When we restrict carbs in our diet, we can prevent pro-inflammatory spikes in blood glucose and blood insulin. Suppression of blood glucose and insulin spikes can be very helpful when managing many chronic diseases."

The ketogenic diet does not produce inflammation in the body, making it a diet which simply allows the body to heal.

Doug Kauffman, who has a television program called *Know the Cause*, is also a proponent of this diet. He calls his diet the *Phase One Diet* and the maintenance diet the *Phase Two Diet*. He has written several cookbooks which can be purchased on my website, www.ibeatcancers.com.

Kauffman stresses that eating organic, free range and wild meats will strengthen the body against disease. He also places a great deal of importance on eating lots of vegetables, but avoiding starchy vegetables.

By strictly avoiding the foods that feed cancer and focusing on a healthy diet to meet my body's nutritional needs, I created the perfect environment for my immune system to heal and to speed me on to restored good health.

I found that as I began to eat from Doug Kauffman's suggested menu, the *Phase One Diet*, I amazingly no longer craved junk food. I did not eat meat during my healing process because Hannah thought meat would slow the healing process. However, I subsequently learned that there is absolutely no problem with eating meat, as long as it is organic, free range or wild. Dr. Cass Ingram recommended eating grass fed beef for anyone battling cancer.

I later learned how vitally important it was to avoid eating anything containing garlic, onions, shallots, leeks, chives, asparagus, all plants from the allium family and to also avoid eating mustard. I learned these foods contained alkylating oils, a type of oils which enable the cancer-causing germ to thrive. Much later on, I came to learn that if I committed to a daily regimen of oxygen therapy, described in Chapter 22, this would eliminate the need to avoid these foods.

The Juice of Wild Oreganol proved to be useful in my battle against breast cancer and eliminated the pinching I was experiencing in my rectum; a tumor was there also.

From reading a book by Dr. Cass Ingram, I learned that the Juice of Wild Oreganol was effective against cancer in the lymphatic system, lymphoma and cancer involving the colon, which includes the mouth, throat, thyroid, esophagus, stomach, and rectum, and will work equally well with cancer of the blood, leukemia. However, I learned cancers in other parts of the body will not respond as well to the Juice of Wild Oreganol, but require different herbal treatments. I have written what I learned about these other cancers in Chapter 4. I also mention in Chapter 4 Dr. Hulda Clark's recommendation for overcoming lung cancer, which includes a protocol of 35% food grade hydrogen peroxide.

CHAPTER 4

Beating Ovarian Cancer

Open thou mine eyes, that I may behold wondrous
things out of thy law. —Psalm 119:18

An entire year passed, and although I achieved amazing results and experienced a speedy recovery, I was still plagued by hot flashes, which resulted in many sleepless nights. As long as I ate as a vegan – no meat, no dairy or eggs and ate hemp seeds as my protein source – I experienced no hot flashes or insomnia, but I had difficulty committing to the vegan lifestyle. As I look back now I realize I was estrogen dominant, but at the time, I had no real understanding of this condition, how dangerous it was or how to alleviate it.

My menopausal symptoms continued, year in and year out. In my quest to relieve myself of the tormenting hot flashes, I very foolishly made the decision to try an over-the-counter menopausal remedy. I knew it was most likely a mistake to do this, but on the outside possibility that I could get some relief, I decided to give it a shot, not knowing what else to do. I was desperate to get some relief from the hot flashes, but apparently not desperate enough to commit to being a vegan.

When I did take the over-the-counter menopausal remedy, I succeeded only in opening Pandora's legendary box. God revealed to me in a dream that I was in trouble, and it had the potential of being on a much larger scale than my first experience with cancer. I began to suffer a painful intermittent pinching sensation in my right ovary. My mother died a gruesome death due to ovarian cancer, so it's somewhat of an understatement when I say

I felt extremely concerned. She complained to me many times during her illness that she felt a pinching sensation in her ovaries.

Although I elected not to see a physician for an official diagnosis, I could easily put the symptoms I was experiencing in my body and the details in the dream together and draw a very logical conclusion. I knew I had developed another hormonal cancer, ovarian cancer. I was also aware that, as a diagnostic tool, a biopsy could serve to release more cancerous cells.

I did, however, see my reflexologist during this time, and while she was massaging my feet, she expressed a lot of concern about the swelling she detected in the area of my foot that correlated to my right ovary. Her concern added to my growing anxiety over the situation. Reflexology is a form of ancient Chinese medicinal foot and hand massage that promotes detoxification of the body, as well as serving as a diagnostic tool which is amazingly accurate.

With this very somber realization of what my reflexologist had detected, in addition to the intermittent pinching I was experiencing, I made a lightening quick decision to go back on my original program with the Juice of Wild Oreganol. However, unlike the victory I achieved in my initial experience with a breast cancer crisis, where I had great success, my symptoms persisted. I got no relief at all. I became alarmed and began scanning through all of the health books I now had at my disposal. I was confident there was a remedy for this kind of cancer; I just had to find it!

It was at this time I began to read Dr. Hulda Clark's book, *The Cure & Prevention of all Cancers*. I ordered the herbal products she listed as a curative in her book by overnight delivery. As soon as the package arrived the following day, I took the herbs. Amazingly, by the end of the day I had stopped experiencing the pinching sensation in my right ovary!

A complete outline of the products I used is listed in Chapter 35. All of these products, including a full array of Dr. Clark's books, as well as the books of others who promote this type of treatment, are available at www.ibeatcancers.com.

I saw my reflexologist a few days later, and she was amazed at how quickly I resolved the swelling in my right ovary which she had previously detected. She could not find any sort of abnormality in my ovaries at all. She wanted to know exactly what I had done. It was at this appointment she told me that any time in the past, whenever she had detected swelling in the ovaries in her middle-aged patients, there had always been a serious complication, namely cancer.

I learned that this powerful herbal combination recommended by Dr. Clark was an effective remedy against all types of cancer, regardless of where the cancer may be located in the body. The herbs are powerful and circulate throughout the system, killing the malignant cells. I learned from Dr. Clark's book that it may take years for cancer to resurface in another region of the body, depending on our lifestyle, but the cells of malignancy are there, and a tumor can rebuild again unless one is aware of how to break the cycle of recurring cancer.

According to Dr. Clark, the herbal germ cleanse will effectively treat every kind of cancer that attacks the body from head to toe, such as brain, bone, ovarian, prostate, lung, liver, pancreatic, uterine, skin and testicular cancer, and sometimes must be used in conjunction with other products in order to be completely effective, namely a hydrogen peroxide solution, in the case of lung cancer, prostate cancer and other cancers.

I learned information regarding the treatment of lung cancer by making an Internet search for lung cancer, hydrogen peroxide and the genius of Dr. Hulda Clark. The person who provided the information in a blog I happened upon stated that it was purely educational information and not medical advice. She spoke of using food grade hydrogen peroxide and distilled water. I have addressed this in Chapter 22.

Dr. Clark wrote about the power of apricot seeds, B17, also known as amygdalin. Amygdalin is recommended in the treatment of lung cancer and other cancers.

I also learned that skin cancer can be treated with good quality hemp oil, applied topically, along with the herbal germ cleanse outlined in Chapter 19 and the diet changes prescribed by Doug Kauffman, author of the Phase One Diet.

I found the herbal germ cleanse remedy recommended by Dr. Clark is also much easier to take, as there is not the strong odor and offensive taste of the wild oregano products.

According to Dr. Clark, the combination of the three herbs in this particular herbal germ cleanse can be safely used even while on medications and will not cause headache or nausea. Dr. Clark said even children can take these herbs, but at much smaller dosages. The recommended dosages for children and pets can be obtained from my website, www. ibeatcancers.com.

I used the Dr. Clark herbal germ cleanse and also took the Juice of Wild Oreganol, just to make sure I eliminated any cancer cells that may have been present in my lymphatic system.

There are many companies that market these herbs, but Dr. Clark said for various reasons, they may be weak and ineffective. According to Dr. Clark, this is largely due to the black walnut hulls being harvested too late in the season; the product's effectiveness may lessen due to issues with storage. In some cases, fillers may be added, making the herbs less potent.

In order to avoid problems with the product's effectiveness or any sort of delay, I would always choose to purchase Dr. Clark's products for myself. I found Dr. Clark's products to be wonderful.

I am sure there are other companies that market excellent products; I am just unfamiliar with them. Dr. Clark said in order to be at all effective, the black walnut tincture should be green. The tincture does not have a long shelf life. I found OW & Company's black walnut tincture is a nice green color, so this would indicate that their product would also be effective.

Dr. Clark recommended that her products be put into the freezer for twenty-four hours before use, except for the tincture which should be refrigerated. Because I live in Florida and have to contend with heat and humidity, I have made a practice of storing Dr. Clark products in a cool, dry cupboard or in my freezer, taking out what I need on a daily basis.

If a person makes the decision to contact the Dr. Clark Store, it is important to remember that federal law prohibits any company from making any claims or dispensing any advice about treating cancer or any other disease. Again, a User Guide for administering the germ cleanse to children and pets is available on my website at www.ibeatcancers.com.

The Dr. Clark Store will email a list of physicians who follow this protocol, meaning recommended methods, upon request. These physicians are located in various regions of the world. Consulting with these individuals can offer support for those who do not choose to go it alone, as I did.

From what I understand, some of the doctors on the list will treat by telephone. Inquiring about a doctor who practices alternative medicine at an independently owned health food store might also prove to be productive.

The principle reason I was able to avoid seeking outside help was that I fully realized the origin of my cancer, estrogen, and I stopped using it. If I had developed cancer and was unable to link the disease with a cause, I would have needed to contact a physician who practices this method of healing. Dr. Clark explained that if one is unable to detect the cause of their cancer and make appropriate changes, the person can fully expect to be placed in the position of a continual tug of war for their health. She stressed a person must be able to identify what it is in their environment that is making them sick and then eliminate it. Dr. Clark stressed over and over again the importance of removing toxins from the environment.

In an interview recorded on an untitled DVD, I watched as Dr. Clark shared the story of a gentleman she treated for lung cancer at her clinic in Mexico. After performing a brief analysis of his blood, she very quickly told him he had an undetected gas leak in his home. As it turned out, the gentleman did indeed have a gas leak in his home. He was healed of cancer by Dr. Clark and has shared his story with many people. I read his amazing story on the Internet.

Unless he had been made aware of the gas leak and fixed the problem, he never would have been able to maintain his good health; instead, when he returned home, he would have relapsed.

In this same untitled DVD, I also viewed an interview of a well-known Italian physician who happened to also be the personal physician to the Pope. He stated that he followed Dr. Clark's method in the treatment of all of his cancer patients and experienced excellent results, saving many lives.

CHAPTER 5

Estrogen Dominance & Breast Cancer

Thy two breasts are like two young roes that are twins,
which feed among the lilies. – Song of Solomon

Although I received remarkable and positive results in my very close brush with stage 4 breast cancer, there was much that I did not yet understand with respect to estrogen dominance. For a woman, estrogen makes the world go round; it is absolutely wonderful! It's what makes her feminine and love life with intensity and passion. On the upside, estrogen is responsible for a woman's passion for her husband, and on the downside, it's most likely the reason her husband is waiting in the car and blowing the car horn while she is finishing her makeup; she wants to look pretty for her husband.

So estrogen serves a purpose. However, an excessive amount of estrogen is lethal. I learned that not every woman has the same level of estrogen. Yes, our age is a factor, but so is heredity. A woman with a high-pitched voice has a higher level of estrogen and her chances of eventually developing hormonal cancer are much higher than that of a woman with a deeper voice.

Although I recognized there was a connection between my breast cancer and the bio-identical estrogen cream I was using, I had no real concept of how heavily permeated my diet and environment was with additional amounts of very harmful estrogens. Like many women, I did not have a clue as to the danger that estrogen dominance posed to my health. I was under the impression that the only real downside to estrogen dominance was that it caused a lot of tension in my marriage every month and added a few extra pounds around my middle. Eventually, I learned that when a person is suffering with a hormonal cancer and there is estrogen dominance, they will NEVER get well unless the estrogen source is eliminated.

I can best describe the naïve state of many of us when it comes to estrogen dominance by telling the story of a woman named Charlotte. Charlotte was a classic example of doing many of the wrong things and getting another chance to remain among the living!

Charlotte learned of me and my experience with breast cancer and my successful outcome through the grapevine of life and made contact with me by email. She requested my telephone number, as she wanted to call and speak with me. Charlotte was battling breast cancer for the second time.

After only a few minutes on the telephone with Charlotte, I was able to quickly share with her my experience and the part estrogen played in my developing breast cancer.

Charlotte told me her story and related to me that she was eating a plentiful amount of non-organic chicken as well as eating her fill of non-organic dairy products. I explained to her the foods she was consuming contained a lot of estrogen and that too much estrogen results in estrogen dominance.

In addition to her diet, I was able to share with Charlotte how our environment can also be a source of estrogen. Her response to me was that her doctor had told her she was estrogen dominant.

Isn't it amazing the oncologist Charlotte consulted with, in an effort to recover her health, would inform her she was estrogen dominant, yet neglect to offer an explanation or a solution to estrogen dominance? Most especially when she was suffering with a hormonal cancer!

I learned that if a woman with hormonal cancer eliminates these dangerous estrogens from her life, she can recover! To withhold this valuable information from a woman with breast cancer is to sentence her to death.

I also shared with Charlotte other things I had learned, such as the fact that non-organic chicken meat is grown with the use of antibiotics and that these antibiotics were passed on to her when she ate the chicken. I had learned that antibiotics actually serve to break down the body's built-in immune system, making a person vulnerable to disease. In Chapter 10, I explain the simple steps I took to strengthen my immune system.

Charlotte told me her story, which included a lumpectomy and the diagnosis of breast cancer three years earlier. The cancer was back again, and she did not understand why it had returned.

I explained what I had learned: We develop cancer as a result of our lifestyles. If the doctor removes the cancerous tumor, and we fail to make changes, we will develop cancer again, plain and simple.

After listening to my experience, Charlotte decided to purchase the same products I used to recover my health. Charlotte's body immediately responded, and a week later, she noticed she began experiencing more of the same symptoms that prompted her to contact me initially, swelling, throbbing and discoloration in her breast.

By this time, Charlotte realized each time she went into her bedroom, her breast started throbbing. Charlotte's body was reacting to the presence of dangerous toxins.

She finally pinpointed the problem as being the fumes from the new carpet which had been recently installed in her apartment. She had the carpet removed and was working on getting well. Charlotte began to focus on removing the harmful estrogens from her diet and toxins from her environment and focusing on rebuilding her immune system.

Charlotte's experience with new carpet during her battle with cancer can be a warning to all of us. Dr. Clark stressed in her book to avoid purchasing any new furniture, to avoid painting or hanging wallpaper and to avoid putting down new carpet while health-challenged because of the toxins. I learned that when I purchase new clothing, I should wash it before wearing it. Likewise, I learned if I bought a new car, I should also purchase an ozonator to remove the new car odor, as the new car odor is comprised of toxic fumes, which are harmful to anyone health-challenged.

From reading Dr. Clark's book, *The Cure & Prevention of all Cancers,* I learned how to either ozonate my non-organic foods to eliminate estrogens or to eat organic meats, organic dairy products and organic produce. I learned about a product called DIM or DIM Plus or a similar product, such as Women's Best Friend, products which remove dangerous estrogens from the body.

Non-organic meats and non-organic dairy products are both dangerous sources of estrogen. Harmful estrogens, known as xeno estrogens, are also present in the non-organic produce we eat and the softened plastics they are packaged in. When eating these foods during the recovery process, I learned to either use an ozonator before preparation, or purchase organic produce. I did not eat exclusively organic vegetables when I battled cancer, as they were not always available to me. Chapter 20 includes the instructions Dr. Clark gave on how to use an ozonator.

I learned to avoid chlorine--which also produces estrogen dominance--by using a showerhead that filters chlorine and by making sure my drinking water was chlorine free alkaline water. Finally, I learned to avoid non-organic cleaning products.

I learned that black cohosh is an estrogenic herb that is dangerous for all those who are estrogen dominant or who suffer with a hormonal cancer. I found that eating soy will also produce estrogen dominance and that even fennel has highly estrogenic qualities. I learned to read labels in order to avoid estrogenic products.

Ozonators, chlorine filtering showerheads, alkaline water dispensers and the supplements mentioned in this chapter are available at www. ibeatcancers.com.

CHAPTER 6

What Prompted My Choice of Treatment

Rest in the Lord, and wait patiently for him: fret not thyself because of him who prospers in his way, because of the man who brings wicked devices to pass.—Psalm 36:7

The day following Hannah's arrival at my door with the healing solution for my breast cancer, I made the decision to get a lymphatic massage at a local spa. It made sense to me that I should do whatever I could to stimulate my lymphatic system, most especially in my breast area. The earliest I could be seen was the next day.

I arrived for the appointment and did my best to prepare the massage therapist before she started the lymphatic massage. When she first saw my breast, the look on her face was absolute shock. I assured her it had actually improved and that the tumor had been much larger and more inflamed two days earlier. I told her I had every confidence it would turn out well. She didn't make any further comment and kept any other observations she may have had to herself. She said by the sense of touch, the lymphatic fluid on the left side of my chest— where the tumor was located— felt completely blocked and very thick. She told me the other side was only a little bit better.

After the treatment, she urged me to drink plenty of water and return in three days to repeat the lymphatic massage procedure. It made perfect sense to me that anything I could do to encourage the free flow of fluid in my lymphatic system was definitely a positive, and I returned as she suggested. It also occurred to me the massage therapist was more than just a little curious as to how my situation was going to play out.

At my follow-up appointment three days later, the massage therapist was nothing short of flabbergasted by how much the breast tumor had decreased in size, exclaiming it was at least the size of a baseball the first time she saw it. She wanted to know exactly what I had been taking and hurriedly left to get a pen and paper so she could write down every detail of the protocol I followed. It was at this point she shared with me her mother had suffered with breast cancer and had undergone a mastectomy. She was in absolute awe as she exclaimed the obvious: I had found the solution for the disease of breast cancer.

I followed up with a few more visits to the spa for the next two and a half weeks until the massage therapist said she could feel a free flow of lymphatic fluid in my body. She could no longer detect any signs of blockage or thickness.

When I first realized I had breast cancer, I listened intently to every word which came out of Hannah's mouth. I followed her instructions to the letter, and I got results very quickly. I wanted to keep my breast; I wanted to live; and I definitely did not want to put my body into the hands of conventional cancer treatment. I had witnessed first hand how conventional medicine ravaged my mother's body. The doctors left no stone unturned, for my mother had the best health care insurance money could buy, and my wonderful husband faithfully paid her pricey insurance premiums.

After sharing my story with an unconvinced family member about my breast cancer experience, she informed me that in order for the cancer to qualify as stage 4, it would have had to metastasize or spread to another part of the body. She informed me I shouldn't claim the cancer was at stage 4. I responded to her by saying I had also experienced a severe pinching and throbbing sensation in my rectum simultaneous to experiencing the throbbing mass in my breast. My colonic hydrotherapist actually saw the tumor on my rectum. What this family member stated about the cancer spreading to another area of the body was a confirmation for me. My cancer was indeed what the conventional medical community would term the final stage, as I had a pinching, throbbing mass in two separate parts of my body.

I recall very well my mother's complaint of the pinching sensation she experienced as the ovarian tumor she suffered with grew larger. I learned from reading *The Cure & Prevention of all Cancers,* by the late Dr. Hulda Clark, that cancer easily spreads or metastasizes, as the cells separate from the mass and move along in the body's lymphatic system and bloodstream. I learned that a blow or bruise to the body can result in the malignant cells travelling to other places in the body.

I know without a doubt people may criticize me for not consulting with a physician or otherwise documenting my breast cancer. But I realized what I had—cancer of the breast caused by too much estrogen. Once I realized the Juice of Wild Oreganol, along with a lifestyle change, would stop the tumor in its tracks, it became unnecessary for me to consult with anyone. What exactly would an oncologist do for me? The medical profession claims they are still searching for the cure.

It's almost beyond belief that the cancer industry is so successful in concealing the simple and inexpensive solution for cancer. Health care drives nearly one fifth of our economy, and the problem is the industry is searching for a cure which will cost a lot of money.

The fact the disease of cancer is spawned by a germ was established by a researcher in the 1940's; this is not new information. Though they may have been ignorant of the fact that cancer was caused by a germ, ancient peoples successfully treated cancer with herbs.

Pharmaceutical companies employ some of the brightest and most well educated people on the planet to research this disease; I would hope so anyway. These people are either simply refusing to acknowledge that God placed an inexpensive answer for cancer in the garden, or they are hiding the fact. This is an industry interested in making a profit. They are not interested in a cheap solution you can follow at home on a shoestring budget!

Bible scripture states in the book of Ezekiel, as well as in the book of Revelation, that the leaves of the trees are for the healing of the nations. This means there is an herbal cure for every degenerative disease known to mankind! What the word of God says is the truth, and we should never

35

forget this is the infallible Word of God, a God who loves people and wants the best for them.

I read that when a woman arrives at the typical cancer treatment center with stage 4 breast cancer, she is given two choices of treatment. She can undergo surgery, chemotherapy, and radiation, and if she is well-insured, she is steered in this direction. If she arrives uninsured and without any source of funds, she is steered in the direction of what is termed supportive or palliative care, meaning there is an acknowledgment the cancer is incurable—too far gone for a cure to even be remotely possible—and her only option is the administration of pain-killing pharmaceuticals, i.e., morphine. She receives a referral to hospice; so hospice can keep her as comfortable as possible as she awaits the inevitable, death.

This would have been a choice given to me. The administration of morphine shuts down the body's organs and results in the patient very quickly losing their desire to live. Morphine administered as pain medication is a death sentence.

I had firsthand knowledge of two women who were diagnosed with breast cancer a few years before I myself developed the disease. Both of these women were beloved friends of mine. One did not survive, and the other one, who had her breast removed, along with a considerable amount of tissue and lymph nodes under her arm and on the side of her body, did survive. I did not personally see her scars, but she described her scarring to me as being "butchered and very ugly."

My friend, who passed away from breast cancer, battled the disease for about three or four years. She had at least three surgeries and took several rounds of chemotherapy as well as radiation treatments. After her preliminary treatment, the cancer was found in her uterus and hip, as well as her brain. Early on in her diagnosis, on more than one occasion, I contacted her at home and encouraged both her and her husband to seek some advice from a physician who practiced alternative medicine and to even search the Internet for alternative approaches to healing cancer.

I didn't know for certain what the natural solution was at this time. However, I was well aware, as the result of watching my mother's battle with ovarian cancer, conventional medicine definitely did not have the answer.

I also urged this couple to visit a health food store—the one Hannah managed. At this time, I was completely unaware of the magnitude of the wisdom Hannah actually possessed. However, my friend and her husband claimed they had it all under control. Her husband said he had a complete plan of treatment mapped out for her recovery. I know for a fact she had the best conventional medical treatment money could buy, as this particular couple was quite wealthy. She even received treatment in another state, having a relative there who was a physician and could recommend one of the state's finest facilities.

The last time I saw this lady, I bumped into her and her husband at the grocery store. I was completely shocked by her appearance. Her health had been completely ruined by the treatments she had received. A once vibrant, energetic, and very athletic person – she could leave me in the dust when we ran together –whose appearance was always stylish, she was now wearing a ragged wig. She had no eyebrows or eyelashes, and her once beautiful smile was weak. She was stooped over, with the appearance of a ninety-year-old woman suffering with a very bad case of osteoporosis. From a layman's point of view, I assumed her appearance of accelerated aging was most likely the result of being administered a pharmaceutical drug designed to pull every speck of estrogen out of the body in order to slow the growth of hormonal cancer. She passed away shortly after I saw her, about two weeks before my own breast cancer surfaced.

As I mentioned previously, in addition to chemotherapy, she also received radiation treatments.

I learned from reading one of Dr. Cass Ingram's books that though tumors do indeed initially shrink as the result of radiation, they always return with a vengeance. The end result of radiation treatment is an increase in the strength of a tumor and destruction of the immune system. The cancerous tumor cells are able to restructure and strengthen themselves against radiation following this type of treatment, so any follow-up radiation has little or no deleterious effect on the cancer cells. This is the point where the treating physician says he has done all he can do. The next thing you know, you are handed a brochure that contains a contact number for your local hospice.

The friend of mine who was horribly scarred and survived a bout with breast cancer, about a year before my breast cancer visibly appeared, endured one round of chemotherapy following surgery. She is a lovely lady from Brazil. My friend's experiences with the side effects of chemotherapy treatments were so horrific she stated she would rather die than go through another round of chemotherapy.

By her husband's own account, she lay on her bathroom floor vomiting blood. Her doctor neglected to write an anti-nausea prescription, and for some reason, the pharmacy was unable or unwilling to contact him over the weekend.

Although her oncologist pleaded with her, promising he would make sure she had the proper anti-nausea medication she needed, promising she would not have a repeat of that terrible experience, she stood firmly and declared she would not be administered any more chemotherapy. She told me she would rather die!

Oddly enough, this awful experience may have ultimately resulted in her survival. When she related her agonizing experience to me, saying she would not and could not repeat another round of chemotherapy and declaring she would rather die of cancer, I gave her the business card of a physician who practiced alternative medicine. I had picked it up from my health food store.

My Brazilian friend called this doctor. As it turned out this physician was married to a Brazilian woman. This gave them common ground, and she felt she could trust his advice. She followed his instructions, changing her diet, and she is now healed, healthy, and beautiful.

The one thing, which really stands out in my mind with regards to this particular lady, was her home environment. It was a lovely, airtight, energy-efficient lakeside home, and there were many giant oak trees surrounding the house, with large branches which shaded her entire roof. Every time I had occasion to visit with her in her home, I noticed I began to get a sore throat. This lady keeps a spotless house, but I observed mildew on the air conditioning ducts of her home, and her husband had mentioned to my husband he had to spray the roof with chlorine periodically to get rid of the heavy mildew accumulation caused by the large oak trees that shaded their entire home, coupled with Florida's high levels of humidity.

After she was diagnosed with breast cancer, I purchased a good quality plug-in air purifier which cleans the air of mildew spores and other impurities and gave it to her as a gift. I suggested she use it in her bedroom, as I had noticed when I visited her home during her illness the mildew odor was strongest in that room, a place where she spent a lot of time. I was unaware of the solution to the disease of cancer at this time, but I was fully aware of the fact that mildew and mold played a role in cancer development. I learned this by watching Doug Kauffman's program, Know the Cause.

Air purifiers are available on my website, www.ibeatcancers.com. The smaller versions of air purifiers are a great item to take along while traveling and staying in hotels or on a cruise!

There is most definitely a link between mold and mildew and developing cancer, and I later learned spraying Oregaspray, also a North American Herb & Spice product, into air conditioning ducts is a safe and effective solution, as the herbal blend in Oregaspray kills mildew and mold. I also learned that using chlorine as a cleaning agent is dangerous, as it is associated with estrogen dominance and is toxic to the body.

Although I had not contemplated what decision I would make if I had developed breast cancer, by mere observation of the health crises these two dear women experienced, I was more than convinced conventional medicine did not have the answer for the disease of breast cancer. Remember, conventional medicine does not even claim to have the cure, only that they are desperately searching for the cure and therefore urgently need more funding.

I saw firsthand the results of the cancer treatments on my own dear mother, who tried her best to have faith and bravely endure the dreadful side effects which inevitably followed such toxic medications. She was horribly sickened by the many treatments of chemotherapy and developed Parkinson's disease as one of the side effects. Her leg would uncontrollably jerk and shake the entire bed; a side effect no one even bothered to mention when initially offering chemotherapy treatment as a lifesaving solution.

My mother wore wigs and scarves to cover her bare head and did her level best to carry on without the slightest complaint. She also underwent several surgeries and required the surgical insertion of three separate ostomy devices to extend her life, which filled with bodily gases and needed almost constant attention. The three ostomy sites and the bags attached to her body at the time of her death were constantly inflamed and leaking gastric juices, burning her already raw skin and causing her tremendous discomfort.

When you have a front row seat to an experience as gruesome and heart wrenching as that was, it has a very sobering impact. When you are providing daily care for a loved one being treated for the disease of cancer, and you are given the grim opportunity to observe the futility of your loved one being subjected to rounds of chemotherapy as so-called curative treatments, painful treatments which do not result in any sort of worthwhile recovery, but rather serve only to contribute to the misery of the illness, it makes a deep impression. It gives you a great deal of hesitation when facing the prospect of being treated for cancer yourself. It should give you cause to think if you have your thinking cap on!

How my dear mother suffered for 4 long years with ovarian cancer and the medical treatments she endured, hoping to recover from the horrible disease or just live a little longer. It was a living nightmare to see my mother—someone who had always been there for me—suffering and in misery. All I could do was try and comfort her, and I did that mostly by buying her lots of beautiful potted orchids in full bloom.

When my mother finally succumbed to ovarian cancer and passed away, it was a great relief to all who loved her. She no longer had to suffer. The spring following her death, I had oodles of blooming orchids to remind me of my awesome mother. My mother was a beautiful Christian woman, and I could now picture her in heaven, a place of peace and happiness.

One night before my mother passed away, while I sat on the edge of her bed, I casually mentioned the possibility of my getting cancer—just an offhand remark that came blurting out of my mouth; nothing I had actually contemplated; it just popped out. She immediately said to me, "Oh, I pray to God neither you nor your sister ever have anything like this."

Later, when I pondered this scene, I realized the words my mother had prayed were very powerful and heartfelt, and God had listened to her supplication in my behalf. God actually did better than my mother's prayers. He did exceedingly and abundantly above all she had asked or thought. He gave me the key to beating cancer and also empowered me to share the affordable solution for cancer with others by writing this book.

Another experience I had which impacted my decision regarding my choice of treatment for breast cancer also involved Hannah. This happened several years earlier, while I still worked as a court reporter.

On this occasion, I worked the entire day at my office without taking time for lunch but instead munched on a couple of peppermint candies I found at the bottom of my purse, and I drank only a few sips from the water fountain in the office. By the time evening rolled around, while I was still at work, the front of both of my legs and the tops of my feet became very swollen, and my legs felt very stiff.

I had never experienced anything like this before. I tried putting my feet up during the next day, but this had absolutely no helpful effect as far as reducing the swelling. I noticed if I ate anything containing sugar, the swelling increased. As days turned into a full week, I still suffered with the condition, and one morning, while I was out walking my dog, I was barely able to make it home after going less than a block because my legs were stiffened by the swelling. This really alarmed me, and I immediately went into the house and called my doctor's office to make an appointment.

My doctor saw me that very day. After taking my vitals, examining me and eyeballing my legs and feet, he told me frankly he didn't have a clue as to what was wrong with me but wanted to start with some tests. The first test he wanted to schedule me for was a circulation test. He told me to schedule the test with his receptionist at the desk. I made the appointment, as he suggested, and left the office, heading for home.

On my way home, I thought, there is nothing wrong with my circulation. My feet look beautiful; they are not discolored, only swollen. I made a quick U-turn and traveled in the direction of the health food store. As soon as I got there, I headed straight for Hannah and showed her my feet. She promptly told me I needed to cleanse my kidneys by eating lots of fresh vegetables, even juicing them if I wanted to, and to stay completely away from grains and sugars as well as any kind of potatoes. Within two days, all of my symptoms totally disappeared. It has now been several years since I had that experience, and the problem never returned.

I may well have had a very different outcome if I had chosen to follow the path of conventional medicine when I initially developed the symptoms with my legs and feet. Besides the tests I may have had to endure, I quite possibly would have been subjected to a myriad of pharmaceuticals and their noxious side effects in my quest for healing.

It was this initial positive experience which led me to conclude Hannah was onto something. Following such great success with this health crisis, every time she delivered my groceries, Hannah dropped off all kinds of information—articles, books, tapes, CDs, and DVDs which contained a wealth of practical information on the natural way to restore your health, and it all made so much sense. She was delighted that someone was open to what she had learned.

From that time on, I began to gravitate toward natural products for any health issues my husband and I experienced. Prior to this, I would visit the local drugstore and buy over-the-counter medications or prescription antibiotics, not even realizing until much later how very dangerous those products can actually be to use. If one of us started sneezing or developed a scratchy throat, I visited a health food store. It was around this time that I began using a North American Herb & Spice product. Their wonderful product Oregaresp should be in every household, rather than the multitude of leftover antibiotics and dangerous over-the-counter medications which now grace a lot of medicine cabinets.

Except for the time I developed a cold when I was recovering from cancer, when I experienced what is termed a healing crisis as a result of the die-off of toxins in my body, I have never developed another full-blown cold. As soon as I have any recognizable symptoms—a sore throat or the sniffles—I take a generous dose of Oregaresp, 3 or 4 capsules, every three or four hours, and all of the symptoms disappear within a day.

I have shared the details of the illness I suffered years ago, along with my experience of nipping colds and sore throats in the bud, in order to give you some insight as to why I had gained such confidence in a natural herbal solution to the throbbing mass in my breast, coupled with my understanding of the dream God had given me.

About one month before I found myself with breast cancer, I injured my knee. I had crawled all of the way from the tailgate into the front seat of my husband's SUV because the electric locking mechanism in his vehicle malfunctioned, and I was otherwise locked out of the car. I made it all of the way to the driver's seat, but as my fanny slid into the bucket seat, my sneaker stuck to the dashboard. My knee twisted, and I heard it rip. It was excruciatingly painful. My knee swelled to nearly twice its size, and I had to lie in bed for a few days while it was packed in ice by my husband. I was still limping from this injury when I realized I had breast cancer.

After I recovered from breast cancer in only 3 weeks, I was still limping from my knee injury. I said to Hannah, "You can heal breast cancer, but you can't fix my knee?"

She replied, "Mary, you just need to take seven or eight Wobenzym and a good-quality, sugar-free noni juice, about an ounce, on an empty stomach every morning." She told me not to drink coffee because the acid prevented healing.

I was back at the gym in two weeks, ready for my Pilates class! Wobenzym are awesome. I found that they eliminated inflammation and scar tissue in my body, as well as supported the formation of healthy tissue. I learned that Wobenzym are enzymes derived from cattle and are most effective for those who have blood type O, as I do, but that other blood types would get better results using plant based enzymes to expedite healing

Following the day which had the potential of being completely terrifying and deadly, but instead ended so beautifully, my husband arrived home each subsequent afternoon wanting a full update on how much the breast tumor had shrunk that day. We thanked God over and over again— not just for my healing, but also for the potential impact my healing would have on other people who were suffering with cancer. We rejoiced knowing we no longer had to fear that we would ever suffer and die with the dreadful disease which had taken the life of my own dear mother.

A man by the name of Anthony Robbins, a renowned motivational speaker, was quoted as saying, "If you do what you have always done, you will get what you have always gotten."

When I faced cancer, suddenly I was where my mother had been ten years earlier. Something inside me—it was the voice of God—told me not to take that same path of treatment which had been of no lasting benefit to my mother, but I would have had no choice but to see a physician if it had not been for my dream from God.

Even after I was fully recovered from breast cancer, I remained absolutely astonished that I recovered so quickly. I said to Hannah, "I'm curious, just how many people have you saved from dying of cancer?"

Hannah's response to me was, "Mary, you are the very first one. No one else would believe me enough to follow through with the protocol. They were all afraid it wouldn't work." Hannah also dropped a bombshell on me when I made the inquiry as to how many other lives she had saved.

Hannah said, "You know what this means, Mary, you have to write a book! You can't keep this to yourself!"

Hannah had learned about the effectiveness of the Juice of Wild Oreganol by chance when she attended an annual health fair in Orlando, Florida, five years earlier. A relative of Hannah's had passed away from pancreatic cancer one month before. Her disappointment with not being able to save their life was still heavy on her heart. As it turned out, a gentleman who was standing near the display of the North American Herb & Spice products was a physician.

Hannah struck up a conversation with the gentleman, and after an extensive discussion and learning he was a doctor, she asked him, "Tell me, and is there a cure for cancer?"

The physician walked over to the display case and picked up a bottle of the Juice of Wild Oreganol and handed it to Hannah. He told her he had experienced outstanding results with the product. He shared with her that he was currently treating a woman with breast cancer with the product, and the woman's breast tumor had shrunk considerably after just one week of taking the product.

Hannah eagerly ordered the product for her store and sold it for the many uses the company was allowed by the FDA to recommend, the treatment of cancer not being one of the allowed recommendations. She held onto that information and the product for five years until I called her for help. Without someone who would actually trust she knew what she was talking about, her hands were completely tied.

What must be understood is the treatment of breast cancer – as well as other types of cancer – is a very profitable business, a multi-billion-dollar business, to be exact. Breast Cancer Awareness Month is little more than a ploy by the cancer industry to promote cancer drugs and a regularly scheduled mammogram—a very dangerous, but lucrative diagnostic test. I did not come up with this summation on my own; I acquired this description of a mammogram from an ob/gyn that practices alternative medicine.

I listened to a radio interview of a well-respected and noted New York oncologist, Dr. Charles Simone. In his interview, Dr. Simone stated emphatically that "screening for breast cancer did not insure an increase in the survival rate of breast cancer victims."

Dr. Simone put great emphasis on this fact, that just because a woman may be vigilant about getting a mammogram, her chances of surviving if a tumor is found in an early stage are not increased at all. This is completely contrary to the message provided by the American Cancer Society.

Dr. Simone also said in order for a woman to decrease her chances of developing breast cancer in the first place, she must reduce the amount of sugars and bad fats she ingests. That is a polite way of telling us that if we don't stop eating so much junk, we are going to kill ourselves!

I then listened to other physicians who practiced alternative medicine who stated that a mammogram utilizes radiation, and radiation is one of the root causes of all cancer.

Therefore, the conclusion they all were drawing was that the more mammograms you have, the greater your chances of possibly developing a breast tumor. What they all agreed on was that a person should utilize a safe method of screening for breast cancer, a digital infrared thermal imaging, which they claim results in a far more accurate diagnosis anyway.

Lastly, Dr. Simone said that the treatment for breast cancer was relatively the same treatment as administered in the 1920s. Here we are in the next century. Does that sound like a race to you?

In reality, the breast cancer industry is marketed with a lot of glitzy advertisement, drawing in well-meaning and compassionate people from all walks of life to run for or walk for the cure while decorating the issue with the color pink at every opportunity. These are somewhat deceptive practices to trick people into thinking the conventional health care industry is interested in making great strides in the race for the cure. What the industry is interested in is great profits. I have read that when a person who has insurance is first diagnosed with cancer, he or she is worth an estimated $500,000 of income for the medical industry.

One source in an article I found on the Internet claimed that in the year 2010, pharmaceutical companies profited a total of $700 billion from the sale of chemotherapy medication alone.

An attorney friend of my husband's, who lost her partner to colon cancer after a 7 year battle, told me his insurance company was billed $36,000 for one single bag of chemotherapy. What on earth could possibly be in one bag of chemotherapy medication which would warrant such an exorbitant cost, especially when it apparently doesn't work, but instead damages the immune system and the body's organs beyond repair?

I do not discount the effectiveness of conventional medicine when it comes to treatment of many ailments. My own husband, who suffered a stroke after drinking over-the-counter cough syrup which elevated his blood pressure, was saved from a premature death by doctors practicing conventional medicine. Seeing a good, well-qualified physician for a yearly exam is wisdom.

When I enthusiastically shared my story of being healed of breast cancer so quickly with my chiropractor, he told me he knew for a fact cancer was easily curable using alternative medicine. He stated that if he ever attempted to help one of his patients employ alternative methods in order to be healed of cancer, the government would not waste any time in pulling his license to practice chiropractic treatments.

The FDA takes a very dim view of many alternative treatments and has placed many restrictions on companies who market these type of products. Lest you may think this is an approach our government has taken only recently, I'll share a true story related to me by a lady I'll call Lucinda. Lucinda's father was diagnosed with leukemia in the 1950's. Being a resourceful gentleman, he located a company through a magazine publication that sent him a monthly mail-order medication which claimed to cure leukemia. Wow, have things changed! The company's claims were indeed bona fide, as he had very nearly made a complete recovery from all of the symptoms of the deadly leukemia when he received a letter from the company, stating the federal government had shut down their operation. Even though he still needed the medication to completely recover from leukemia, he was able to live out a normal lifespan by avoiding toxins the company had linked to the disease.

I have heard it said of more than one oncologist—a specialist in treating cancerous tumors--they absolutely would not undergo chemotherapy treatments if they were ever diagnosed with cancer. An acquaintance of mine recently shared a story with me about a friend of hers who has practiced oncology for years. He was suffering with an inoperable brain tumor and checked himself into an alternative medicine clinic.

Oncologists are very intelligent people, and they are well aware of the shortcomings of their methods, that in most instances, one may actually live longer, and enjoy a better quality of life, if they forego conventional treatment and adopt a healthy lifestyle.

Another reason the cure for cancer eludes society is probably the most astounding of all and really has made a broad entrance for the questionable methods of cancer treatment. As a society, we do not want to take personal responsibility for our health. A person would be hard-pressed to watch television or listen to radio or Internet programming and not hear some expert speaking on what part an unhealthy lifestyle plays in the diagnosis of cancer. Yet most people turn a deaf ear to this advice for one astonishing reason: They simply do not want to change their lifestyles. They choose to eat processed foods that not only offer very little nutrition, but also contain germs and harmful, addictive ingredients which are toxic to their bodies.

People very often do not seem to care about the toxins they ingest daily until they encounter a crisis situation. Processed foods leave a person drained of energy, as they offer very little nutritional support to the body. When people have no energy, they don't exercise. When the body is not exercised, there is an insufficient flow of oxygen, which in turn serves to further weaken the immune system. Processed foods can set the body up for disease. What seems to be an inexpensive, fast and convenient source of food can eventually lead to the development of a disease. Disease in turn costs our government great amounts of money to try and remedy in the way of federal spending on health care. What a vicious cycle!

In short, people choose to ignore sound advice and take what they perceive to be the easy way out; they choose to just eat what is convenient, rather than taking the time to prepare healthy food. The result of paying no heed to the necessity of good nutrition creates a nation of people with poor health. This lifestyle of poor eating habits adversely affects human initiative and even impairs a person's ability to think decisions through logically. Our brains require good nutrition to function well. When our diet does not provide good nutrition, we are void of physical energy. Poor nutrition can produce an individual who will complacently allow others to make decisions for them; they relinquish their right to make informed choices for their own health care and blindly trust what can often be very greedy people.

Modern medicine boasts that they have made breakthroughs treating certain types of cancer, but at what cost? There are a multitude of cancer survivors who received chemotherapy and have sustained permanent damage to their vital organs. They cannot expect to live out a normal lifespan with damage to their vital organs. Can that really be considered a breakthrough in medicine?

When I was first healed of breast cancer, I was just brimming with enthusiasm about the natural approach for the cure of cancer. I shared my story with nearly everyone I engaged in conversation. Many people shared with me that although they did not know what the solution was, they were positive there had to be a natural approach which was possibly more effective.

As a society, we have been so conditioned to think that for a cure to be viable, it must be very costly, even financially out of reach to the uninsured. How could the cure for cancer be so simple? Doesn't it require expensive pharmaceuticals and equally expensive treatments with special equipment? The tool, which is used to prevent so many from taking a natural approach to cure cancer, is fear. When anxiety rules the day, the human mind loses its ability to think logically.

Dr. Lorraine Day addressed this in her book about being healed of breast cancer naturally, simply by changing her diet. She documented her cancer by taking a photo, and I saw the picture of her breast, which showed a tumor about the size of a plum growing out of her chest. It took her months of proper eating to achieve healing. She did not even have the benefit of the knowledge of the fast acting anti-cancer herbal germ cleanse or the amazing little apricot seeds I mention or the knowledge of 35% H202, yet she was able to heal herself through diet.

Dr. Day tells people not to be afraid or to allow conventional medicine to bully them into making a quick decision. To quote Dr. Day, "The tumor you have has very likely been there for years. When you are diagnosed with cancer by a physician, it is very often not an emergency. You have time to make an informed decision. You have time to utilize a proven alternative treatment."

Make a decision with some age-old wisdom in mind—a quote from Hippocrates. "Let food be thy medicine, and let medicine be thy food." Hippocrates also said, "Walking is man's best medicine." Being active has an extremely positive effect on our health!

Make an informed and quality decision based on fact rather than just assuming there are no other options. You do not have to die a premature death! You can live and be so chockfull of vitality and enthusiasm that you inspire others!

Allow this simple book to provoke you into thinking for yourself! Locate a doctor who is willing to work with you by requesting a list of doctors who practice this type of medicine from the online website of the Dr. Clark Store.

CHAPTER 7

Testimonies

I would have fainted, unless I had believed
to see the goodness of the Lord in the land
of the living.—Psalm 27:13 NIV

I crossed paths with some people who were desperate to be healed of cancer. Although some were insured, they were reluctant to subject themselves to the methods of conventional medicine, usually after witnessing firsthand the poor results that a family member or close friend experienced or having suffered themselves with previous cancer treatments which proved to be both ineffective and debilitating.

I also crossed paths with some people who were financially desperate and uninsured. One person who knew me from church simply believed me enough to try the method I used rather than first seeing a surgeon. They were all healed!

The first lady I was able to help was an older woman in her late 60's; we attended the same church. She was prescribed estrogen as a vaginal cream by her doctor—not a good idea. Maybe she talked her doctor into giving her the estrogen cream against his good judgment; I don't know. The end result of her using the estrogen cream was she very soon developed a tumor about the size of a large marble in her vaginal canal. Her doctor referred her to a surgeon.

She called me at home the day after she heard my astonishing healing testimony at our monthly women's meeting at church. She anxiously asked if I thought the alternative treatment I had such great results with would work for her as well. I told her she could give it a try and shared the name of the product. She called me a week later and told me the tumor was completely gone.

After I was healed, I was eager to return to one of my very favorite locations, the gym, where I met up with a beautiful lady by the name of Gail. We frequently worked out together. I explained my recent absence by sharing my amazing breast cancer story with her. Gail, a blue-eyed, blond powerhouse who flipped houses for a living and did roofing jobs on the side, confided in me she had developed a blister inside her nostril which she had attempted to heal for months with rounds of antibiotics she was able to scrounge up, but to no avail. With the downturn in the economy, she had become too impoverished to see a doctor and felt desperate.

Once Gail brought her condition to my attention, I could easily see that the end of her nose was crimson and taking on a purplish undertone, the exact same colors I saw on my breast. She confided in me that she was pretty sure she had cancer in her nose. She had been a real sun worshiper in her youth. Not having any health insurance, Gail decided she was definitely going to try the simple and natural approach I was so enthusiastic about. Within a week, the large blister inside of her nose she had battled for several months was totally gone, and her nose returned to its normal color.

Gail told me one of the reasons she was so open to trying the natural approach first, aside from being uninsured and not wanting to more than likely face a disfiguring surgery anyway, was because her uncle was healed of cancer at a clinic in Mexico. He was an invalid when he was taken to the clinic, and a couple of days following his return home, he went deer hunting. So Gail knew there were options, but she was too broke to go to Mexico. She decided to give the product a try and ended up with amazing results.

I was able to help several other people with this method, but the one who really stands out in my mind is a young woman in her late twenties. She had five young children and was attending a local beauty school in my city.

I had this crazy idea about getting a weave. A weave is created when a stylist neatly braids your hair snugly to the scalp and then sews purchased human hair into the braids, leaving the wearer with thick, long, beautiful hair that initially belonged to someone else. This desire, understandably, irritated my regular hairdresser, who tried to talk me out of what proved shortly thereafter to be a complete numskull of an idea, but I could not be persuaded otherwise.

It turned out my hairdresser's family owned a beauty school, and she gave me the name of a young woman who was presently enrolled at the school and practiced this technique on a regular basis. So I called and made an appointment with Gwendolyn Huntsman (not her real name). This turned out to be truly providential.

Gwendolyn was pleasant as she braided my shoulder-length hair snugly to my scalp and filled me in on what the procedure entailed and how long it would be before it became necessary to tighten the weave. She admired the lovely, long red locks that I had purchased at Silky's Hair Supplies and told me how foxy I would appear to my husband.

When Gwendolyn finished securely sewing the beautiful red locks into my braided hair, I thought it looked fabulous, and I was thrilled with the results. I was sure that my husband would want to take me out to dinner when he got home from the office and let me show off my new "do," even though it wasn't Friday or Saturday night, our usual weekend date nights.

Gwendolyn sweetly smiled and handed me a rattail comb on my way out the door, declaring she had a little gift for me.

My husband's reaction wasn't quite what I had envisioned. He walked in the door, and I gave him a great big smile. He surprised me by returning my foxy gaze with a stern expression on his face, very similar in appearance to the facial expression he had the day I backed my brand-new car -- which was equipped with a back-up camera -- into the garage door after two weeks of ownership. He was not at all impressed, pronouncing with a scowl that he liked my real hair better.

I, however, was completely unfazed by his negative reaction; I loved my glamorous new hairstyle and repeatedly checked myself out in every mirror in the house. Except for my pale complexion, I imagined myself looking very much like one of the sexy Ikettes, who were popular in the '70's, with their long hair weaves, dancing and singing backup in the Ike and Tina Turner Revue! I was "Proud Mary, turnin', burnin' and rollin' on the river."

However, nighttime approached, and it came time for me to lay my head down on my pillow. My elation with my stunning new do took a quick nosedive. My body was relaxed, but my scalp was not able to follow suit, and it itched. As blues vocalist B. B. King used to wail to his audiences, "The thrill is gone."

I lay there, feeling as though a faux fur bathroom rug had been sewn to my head, and I was unable to get it off. I stifled the desire to scream, determined to at least enjoy my sexy new hair long enough to get my money's worth, as I had plunked down quite a chunk of change at Silky's Hair Supplies. I was not about to complain in front of my husband! I turned out the light and quietly fumbled around the bedside table for the rattail comb Gwendolyn had given me.

A couple of weeks passed, and I had all I could take of what had now become my hairdo from Hades. I was more than a little anxious to see Gwendolyn so she could remove the grisly hair transplant. My scalp had become so itchy, I felt as though I had a tiny wild animal crawling around on my skull, and I was unable to exterminate the creature. The weave had shifted and taken on a lumpy appearance, most likely due to my relentless digging and poking at it with the rattail comb which had become my constant companion. I now was forced to wear either a scarf or a hat whenever I left the house. My husband didn't make any comments, but I caught him out of the corner of my eye looking warily at it a couple of times, and he had not touched my head since I had made the acquisition.

I quickly got dressed one Monday morning after he left for his office and headed for the beauty school, but to my dismay Gwendolyn was not there that day. The same thing happened the following day. On the second day, I anxiously spoke with Gwendolyn's instructor about her absence, and she confided in me that Gwendolyn was home sick as the result of a chemotherapy treatment she had undergone for thyroid cancer.

Well, that was all I needed to hear to get my engines fired up. I began relentlessly texting Gwendolyn for the next few days until I finally got a response. She was very ill from the chemotherapy treatment and was forced to take the week off from beauty school to recuperate. I texted her to call me the day she returned to school because I wanted to talk to her, not mentioning my healing testimony. There was no way I would let this girl die and leave that thing stuck on my head. I am sure Gwendolyn had to laugh while she was lying there in her bed, thinking, "I feel like I'm dying, and that crazy white woman wants the weave off of her head!"

Within just a few minutes of her call letting me know that she was back at the beauty school, I arrived with a very unsightly headful of red hair. I shared my dramatic story of being healed of breast cancer with Gwendolyn while she removed the weave, and she, in turn, related her current health crisis.

Gwendolyn told me she had been diagnosed with thyroid cancer by a physician at the same prestigious cancer center I was initially referred to by my doctor's office. She was taken to the local hospital emergency room by her husband when she developed difficulty swallowing and was given a referral to the cancer treatment center after some initial testing at the local hospital. The treating oncologist at the cancer treatment center prescribed three rounds of chemotherapy, after which they would see where she was with regard to the tumor, if the thyroid had shrunk to a small enough size to allow removal by surgery. She had completed only the first round of chemotherapy at the time of our conversation.

Gwendolyn said she would definitely be interested in trying out the natural remedy that had worked so effectively for me. I also shared with her what I ate, focusing on fresh vegetables. I explained that eating the wrong thing would set a person up for failure, that it was important to avoid sugars, fruits, grains, potatoes, breads, and bad fats. This was the diet I followed to be healed of breast cancer.

When my husband came home from his office that evening and saw the rug was missing from my head, and that I had returned to my former hairstyle, he shouted, "Hallelujah!" He put his arms around me and assured me he loved my hair just the way it was and he thought I had beautiful hair. He asked me to please never do anything like that again. Pulling me even closer, he gave me an amorous glance and said, "Hey, why don't we have a romantic dinner tonight at the restaurant of your choice?" Hallelujah! It wasn't even the weekend!

The following week, after having taken the Juice of Wild Oreganol 3 times a day for several days, Gwendolyn went back to her oncologist for her second round of scheduled chemotherapy treatment. Because they were unable to feel or palpate the tumor, which had previously been so large she had difficulty swallowing, there was a decision made to take a biopsy. Less than an hour after the biopsy, her completely astonished oncologist came into the examining room and declared that he had never seen anything like it in his entire career. The lab was unable to detect one single cell of cancer in her biopsy, and she was healed! She was absolutely cancer-free.

This young mother got a new beginning in life. She shared with me later she had told her husband to prepare himself for a future without her. She also added with a big smile that her entire Christian family had prayed God would heal her and allow her to raise her children, the youngest being an infant. Amazingly, God ordered my steps right to her—truly providential!

Does God have a sense of humor or what? Who would have thought my getting a weave was an idea generated by Him? "But God hath chosen the foolish things of the world to confound the wise; and God hath chosen the weak things of the world to confound the things which are mighty" (1 Corinthians 1:27 KJV).

Afterward, Gwendolyn was so grateful and she offered me free weaves any time. No thank you, darling Gwendolyn.

Gwendolyn friended me on Facebook, letting me know she opened her own beauty shop. I "liked" her page, and she responded back. I was very happy for her. She is a real go-getter, and she got a new opportunity to go forward in life with her beautiful family.

Another instance of my being able to help someone was when I was contacted by one of my husband's clients, Marina Yeveg (not her real name.) Marina and her husband, Sergey, who are Russian immigrants and extremely proud of their US citizenship, were referred to my husband about a legal matter. Marina is employed by the judicial system as an interpreter, and she is pretty, extremely bright, industrious and full of love. Her handsome husband, Sergey, also a hard worker, has his own business and spends his spare time coaching their daughter, a budding tennis star.

While at my husband's office, Marina broke down and cried, telling him her legal situation was even more stressful because of her current health problems. She had undergone a radical mastectomy, which included removal of lymph nodes under her arm due to breast cancer, and she suffered serious complications. My husband shared my experience with her, and not long after that, we were able to meet. When I first saw Marina, I could not help but notice how grotesquely swollen her arm appeared—not only a sign of lymphatic blockage, but could also signal the return of cancer.

Marina shared with me she experienced a lot of pain and discomfort in her arm due to the swelling in her lymphatic system, as her body was unable to properly drain the lymphatic fluids since undergoing extensive surgery. In addition to being very painful, it served as a constant reminder that, very probably, deadly cancer cells were lurking around in her body, ready to strike somewhere else.

Marina followed the course of action I shared with her and got excellent results very quickly. The swelling completely left her arm as well as the accompanying pain and soreness. She shared with me she had tried many different treatments and purchased various pieces of expensive medical equipment designed to help reduce lymphatic fluid buildup, making every possible effort to get rid of the painful swelling. She had invested a lot of money into these remedies, and nothing had worked.

She rejoiced, knowing that she had a new lease on life. While enjoying the peace of good health, she was able to delight in her busy role as an interpreter, wife, and mother, and finish the task of raising her youngest child, as well as welcoming her very first grandchild into the family, a precious baby boy named Brian. Marina asked me to also share that my husband won her case!

Another amazing testimony is the healing of Gavin McNamara, (not his real name). Gavin contacted me after being given my telephone number by a mutual acquaintance I will refer to as Janice. Janice and Gavin had struck up a casual friendship while taking the same class at a nearby school. In a conversation during a class break, Gavin mentioned he had survived a bout with lymphoma, and the disease was currently in remission. Janice's response to this was she knew someone who healed herself of cancer using a natural remedy.

Several weeks after hearing this claim from Janice, Gavin began to experience lethargy, and his wife, Jill, who worked in the medical field, was able to feel a tumor in his neck. He returned to his physician, and after undergoing testing, he was told the lymphoma was back—but this time, it had returned with a vengeance. His physician gave him three weeks to live and wanted to commence immediately with an aggressive chemotherapy treatment.

Despite the urgent warning, which came with the doctor's diagnosis, Gavin dragged his feet when it came to submitting to more chemotherapy. His initial experience with undergoing chemotherapy treatments for lymphoma was dreadful. According to Gavin, he had very narrowly survived and was left completely drained of energy. He seriously weighed in his heart whether further treatment would even be effective, as the disease had returned with an even greater onslaught. In addition to this, Gavin had a cousin in Baltimore, who had recently died of the same type of lymphoma with which he had been diagnosed. Coupled with the news of his cousin's death and the fact he had barely survived the earlier treatment, Gavin drew the conclusion that any further chemotherapy treatment was futile. He recalled Janice mentioning she knew someone who healed herself of cancer naturally, and he felt he had nothing to lose by choosing an alternative method.

Gavin made the valiant effort to haul his sick body out of bed the following Monday morning and go to the school, hoping Janice was in class that day, as she had been out herself during a hospitalization. She was there, and as soon as class was over, he approached Janice and disclosed he had just found out the cancer was back and in a more aggressive form than before. Janice gave him my telephone number, and he called immediately.

I briefly shared my experience with Gavin, and Gavin shared his situation with me. As a result of the extensive reading I had done, after just a brief conversation, I was able to tell Gavin exactly why he had developed lymphoma. I told him that he wore a lot of cologne, giving entrance to the solvent isopropyl alcohol into his body, and that he ate a lot of shrimp, a food that will surely take a toll on the health, as it contains allergens and is a trigger food for lymphoma. Gavin told me I was exactly right about both of these two habits he had, and he was completely shocked I knew these two things without ever meeting him.

Gavin made the decision to follow through with the same steps I took, and he and his wife were amazed at his recovery. Three weeks after his doctor's grim prognosis, Gavin underwent another PET scan at his doctor's office. His doctor was unable to find any cancerous cells in his body and declared Gavin was completely healed. His doctor was astonished.

Gavin and his wife came to my home for a visit about a week after we first spoke. During that time, we chatted about various things, among them being how God speaks in dreams. I shared with Gavin's wife Jill how my healing came about as the result of a dream from God. This exchange jogged her memory, and she shared a strange dream with me she had just a few days before Gavin learned of an alternative treatment.

Jill dreamed there was a lamp in their bathroom that began to grow brighter and brighter; she just shrugged it off as a nonsense dream. She marveled when I told her that God is likened to a lamp, bringing the covenant of peace, illumination, wisdom, and knowledge; that a bathroom is a place of cleansing; and that the path of the just grows brighter until the perfect day! Jill's dream was a message from God and revealed He had plans to heal Gavin.

The last I heard from my friend Janice with regard to Gavin, he and his wife planned on spending part of their summer in Europe. Bon voyage, and God bless!

Lastly, I want to share the story of a very spunky lady I will call Jean. Jean is employed at the local supermarket I shop at every week, and she has great health insurance. She had learned of my successful bout with breast cancer through my massage therapist.

Jean approached me one morning at the supermarket after finding a large lump in her breast. She described it as a large knot-like tumor sticking out of her chest, but not inflamed as mine had been. Her physician wanted to do a needle biopsy, but she refused. She had a friend who had suffered with breast cancer, and even though she survived, Jean said she had endured a nightmare of treatment. She also related to me that her friend was still taking a small dose of chemotherapy every day, and the thought of taking chemotherapy treatments was frightening to her. She was reluctant to take any sort of remedy.

I told her to absolutely avoid eating any vegetable in the allium family and mustard. I stressed to her the importance of avoiding isopropyl alcohol and chlorine. I told her what product I used, as well, but she said she was busy and couldn't be bothered. Within two weeks, Jean told me the tumor had shrunk significantly. Jean then went on an Internet search and happened upon a website which recommended amygdalin, a product made of apricot seeds, in capsule form. Months have passed and she no longer has a breast tumor. Now, that was healing on a shoestring budget!

I tried taking amygdalin but, unfortunately, it made me feel nauseated. I think my intolerance to amygdalin is most probably related to my blood type, which is O. I later asked Jean what her blood type was, but she was clueless. I think whether or not a person can tolerate amygdalin may depend on their blood type.

CHAPTER 8

No Fear

For God has not given me a spirit of fear; but of power,
and of love and of a sound mind. —2nd Timothy 1:7

One of the principal keys to my amazing recovery was not allowing myself
to be overwhelmed by fear, but instead putting my trust in God when
He spoke to me in a dream. I allowed His presence to keep me in peace.
Believe me when I say I cannot take any credit for the peace I experienced.
It was all HIM!

Fear has a paralyzing effect on the mind and hinders the ability to
think clearly and rationally, and even more importantly, it hinders our
ability to hear God's voice, which is so often a gentle whisper.

If we heard a noise during the night and found a robber trying to get
into our home, we wouldn't invite him in and fix him a sandwich. Of
course not, instead we would shout, "You, get out of here!" We would use
a weapon against him and call 911, and this is precisely what our response
should be when fear comes to intimidate us; we should not entertain a
spirit of fear.

Dr. Lorraine Day, the physician I mentioned earlier, who healed herself
of breast cancer and wrote a book about the experience, says something
along these lines: The cancer did not appear there overnight, and more
than likely it is not an emergency. In other words, you have time to
make a rational decision. Dr. Day frankly states that the only solution
conventional medicine has as a treatment is to cut, burn and poison. I
am sure you will agree with me none of those options sound particularly

appealing. Can we really expect to get well by poisoning and burning the body? Does that really make any sense?

Conventional medicine's blatantly unsuccessful approach to treating cancer, chemotherapy and radiation, destroys the body's immune system, its built-in healing mechanism. Once you have made a choice of treatment that destroys the immune system, getting well then becomes a much greater challenge. The body cannot get well unless the immune system is functioning properly. If the immune system is shot, all the medicine in the world would fail to heal the body.

A very simplified explanation of the function of B-cells and T-cells is they heal and protect the body from disease; B cells and T-cells have offspring. These tiny offspring have memory and go about policing the body and attacking any foreign substance that may be launching an invasion on our good health. Due to their profound built-in ability to remember exactly what it takes to kill a particular invader, they are able to quickly respond and attack any foreign substance.

This is the reason we don't re-catch the same cold we gave to a family member; the offspring remember what it takes to boot out the cold and quickly overwhelms these intruding germs, thus protecting our body.

Chemotherapy and radiation destroys B-cells, T-cells and their precious offspring that protect our body. The end result of killing these offspring very simply means the body forgets how to heal. The miracle is people are sometimes able to survive this type of medical treatment. Surviving this type of treatment is nothing more than a display of how very strong the body actually is; if you have previously been treated with chemotherapy and radiation, and the cancer has returned, you can get well. Your body can rebuild! Our God made a wonderful and resilient vessel! Remember, the Bible says that with God, all things are possible! God still intervenes in hopeless situations and heals! Read Chapter 10 which explains a simple method on how to rebuild the immune system.

Along with the motivating force of a throbbing tumor the size of a baseball, the speed with which I began to recover when I took the natural approach served to add the momentum necessary to inspire me to make some positive changes in my lifestyle. Translation: I was highly motivated to stop eating junk!

To my utter astonishment, within just a few hours, I had improved significantly, and this served to greatly encourage me to go forward with the natural approach. I discovered ridding the cancer cells from my body could be accomplished simply with herbs which were readily accessible, and I was elated, as well as greatly relieved, to learn I could get well without resorting to the drastic measures employed by conventional medicine.

I then began the process of learning about the many different and powerful detoxification tools which could be employed to aid in recovering from cancer, as well as preventing the disease. I learned I should use a showerhead which filtered chlorine. I also learned that my drinking water needed to be free of chlorine, and I found out there were wonderful benefits from drinking 35% food grade hydrogen peroxide with juice or distilled water. Eliminating chlorine allowed my immune system to rebuild and fight the disease of cancer.

I learned about an ozonator, a wonderful tool which effectively destroys toxins in food and removes toxins from the home environment. I discovered how the awesome ion cleanse foot detox bath cleansed my body of impurities and helped eliminate pain. I learned how a good quality plug-in air purifier would protect me against fungus, mold and mildew in the home, a great item for travel. I found out how wonderfully effective a far infrared sauna was for detoxification, actually killing germs and viruses. These products are available on my website, www.ibeatcancers.com.

I learned of an inexpensive far infrared pad which is amazing in its ability to relieve the body of pain, and the far infrared pad is an excellent item to pack for travelling. I even learned of an energy frequency machine which could be used to help eliminate pain, based on the art of reflexology.

There is a host of effective items from which to choose.

Even though I did not have chemotherapy, I learned of products which would be of benefit to those who make these treatment choices. Dr. Cass Ingram, President of the North American Herb & Spice Company, recommends the use of several of his products to enhance the effects of chemotherapy, as well as preventing the tissue damage caused by chemotherapy and I have included this information in Chapter 35.

Dr. Hulda Clark, author of *The Cure & Prevention of all Cancers*, wrote that an herbal germ cleanse may be safely taken by those who are presently being administered traditional cancer treatment without fear of complications.

Just as in the case of Gwendolyn Huntsman, whose story I wrote about in Chapter 7, these products can give a person the edge when treating with conventional medicine. Gwendolyn incorporated a natural remedy in conjunction with chemotherapy, and after only one chemotherapy treatment, she was declared cancer free.

In her book, Dr. Clark placed a great deal of emphasis on change, stressing the importance of cleaning up our environment and changing the way we cook and the foods we eat in order to remain healed.

For example, I found I could very easily get rid of the cancer, but if I returned to the same lifestyle, eating the wrong foods, such as non-organic meats and dairy products laden with estrogen and antibiotics; grains and sugars; the same toxic cleaning products which promote estrogen dominance; the same chemically laden hygiene and beauty products; all of which played a role in my developing cancer initially, my future would definitely hold another battle with cancer.

SECTION 2

Cancer Causes

CHAPTER 9

The Cause of Cancer

Call unto me, and I will answer you, and
show you great and mighty things which you
do not know.—Jeremiah 33:3 NIV

Through the years Hannah had accumulated a great deal of information about curing disease using alternative medicine, in the way of books, DVDs, and CDs, but because of her hectic work schedule, she was too exhausted to read the material. So she began to make it a habit of sharing information with me. Every time she delivered my groceries she would have a box of books or an armful of pamphlets and other information. I might have just stored all of the information away and gone on with my busy life, but a pinching pain in my right ovary prompted me to start digging even deeper through all of the material she had brought to my house. What I found in the books was not only other herbal cures for cancer, but also an explanation as to why a person develops cancer in the first place.

I learned the disease of cancer is very simply caused by a germ, a germ which produces life-threatening bacteria. A malignant tumor is comprised of this cancer-causing germ, the bacteria it produces, fungus from eating a diet of too many refined carbohydrates, and toxins we have absorbed from commercial hygiene products and our environments in general. In the case of a hormonal cancer such as I had, breast cancer and ovarian cancer, estrogen was the biggest factor. I learned that cancer is not always the result of one particular thing; rather cancer is the result of a combination of factors.

Our body can very easily be compared to a sponge which soaks up whatsoever is surrounding it, as it absorbs anything in the environment, whether it is good for us or whether it is bad for us.

The body has its own built-in detoxification system. However, our modern environments have become so chock full of polluting toxins that our body can become overwhelmed by these toxins and unable to completely cleanse itself. What this means to us is our body is storing toxins.

The changes we experience as the result of storing toxins can be very subtle, so we may even fail to notice the slight difference in our health, just a very, very gradual loss of energy. Eventually, the body, limited by its own natural ability to detoxify all of these noxious substances, becomes overwhelmed with toxins and is simply unable to naturally rid itself of this toxic overload.

When we eat non-organic meats, dairy products and eggs, we are also consuming the estrogens, antibiotics and other medications with which these animals have been treated with or fed. The animals raised for market are not necessarily fed antibiotics because they are sick; rather, they are fed antibiotics because the administration of these pharmaceutical drugs causes the animals to grow larger in size and gain greater body mass. Whatever substance these animals have been fed or injected with by the rancher is passed on to the consumer. If the effect of ingesting these antibiotics makes the animals larger and heavier, you can be sure they will have a similar effect on human beings.

Purchasing organic, free range and wild meat is more expensive. However, when you realize just what you and your family are being protected from by choosing to purchase organic, free range and wild meat, you can easily understand it is a small price to pay to protect your health and the health of your loved ones.

When we take medications, over-the-counter as well as prescription medications and most especially antibiotics, these also contribute to the breakdown of our health. Antibiotics weaken the body's immune system, the very built-in wall of defense that protects the body from disease.

When we consume toxins over a period of years, the body through the circulatory system shoves the toxins together in an attempt to push them out, actually forming a tumor. I learned through my research a tumor is simply a composition of foreign substances the body is attempting to get rid of, but can find no natural outlet.

As the result of the toxic overload, the body is weakened, but there is not yet a malignancy. The reason a benign or non-cancerous tumor becomes malignant or cancerous is due to the cancer-causing germ. This germ has 6 stages and, except for perhaps its last stage, cannot even be seen by the naked eye. I learned the final and rapid process of developing a malignant tumor is greatly accelerated when isopropyl alcohol is present. Isopropyl alcohol enables the cancer-causing germs to multiply at an alarming rate.

I learned that in order to be healed and remain healed, I had to avoid the use of the solvent isopropyl alcohol. I do not understand the connection, but there is a link between isopropyl alcohol and heart disease, as well. I found if I used any product containing isopropyl alcohol on my skin, most particularly on my face and chest, the result would be that in less than an hour my heart would begin pounding wildly.

A couple of years after I realized there was a connection between isopropyl alcohol and this rapid or racing heartbeat, I met a teller at my bank who just happened to mention to me that her husband was having a problem with his heart pounding wildly. She was extremely concerned and said she was going to take him to see a cardiologist. I mentioned my experience with using isopropyl alcohol caused a similar reaction and asked her what hygiene products he was using. She gave me a bewildered stare and gradually began telling me his daily routine, which did include the use of products containing isopropyl alcohol. I spoke with her a couple of months later, and she told me he had had no further episodes after they had eliminated the use of any products containing isopropyl alcohol.

We are all very often frequent users of manufactured beauty products, i.e., hair dyes, make-up, beauty potions, lotions, creams, gels, sprays, soaps, perfumes, mouthwashes, toothpastes and household cleaning products, and all of these items introduce even more toxins into the body.

The task of cleansing the body of toxins and breaking down a tumor must be accomplished in order to fully restore health. Unburdening the body of toxins by cleansing the colon, kidneys, gall bladder, and liver accomplishes this.

Avoiding further contact with toxins or greatly reducing the load of toxins the body is exposed to will then allow for the immune system to be strengthened, and the immune system is then free to carry out the task for which it was created—namely, fighting disease and promoting health and energy.

The methods used to recover from cancer which are outlined in this book are not newly found information, but instead a form of medicine practiced by ancient peoples who recognized the necessity of periodically cleansing the body. These people made it a practice to cleanse seasonally. The Iroquois Indians of North America used the very same herbal germ cleanse recommended by Dr. Hulda Clark. In fact, I heard Dr. Clark's neighbor, an elderly woman of American Indian ancestry, related this curative method prescribed by Dr. Clark.

Now, all disease-generating substances enter the body from the outside in, through toxins, germs, and bacteria. I learned the body does not produce disease on its own accord; the body is actually a sterile vessel. Normally, when we ingest germs, they go through the body and exit in the stool. However, germs are able to access the body through perforations in the gut: One way these perforations occur is through tiny abscesses in the colon created by the germs, which produces a condition called leaky gut, a condition which is far more prevalent than may be realized. I learned that ultra-pasteurized milk causes perforations in the gut, thus producing leaky gut. This shocked me because I was drinking ultra-pasteurized organic milk and thinking I was promoting my good health! Perforations in the gut accelerate the disease process, as it allows cancer-causing germs access to our sterile vessel.

In spite of this, I learned all is not lost, as once the body's contact with these germs and toxic substances are eliminated, and the body is cleansed and detoxified, the body will then be allowed to heal, as the body was created to do, to naturally heal.

When a toxic foreign substance remains in the body, the body is unable to completely heal; the body tries to reject it or shove it out so that it is free to heal. The ability of the body to shove out a foreign substance is the reason a patient who has received a donated organ is required to take anti-rejection medication the remainder of his life, because the body naturally rejects the organ.

We have most likely all experienced a similar situation on a very small scale when we may have gotten a tiny splinter of wood in our finger; the area becomes inflamed as the white blood cells go to work trying to push the splinter out. When the splinter is removed, the finger heals.

This is a very simple illustration, but it is a powerful fact to remember when pursuing good health. Eliminate the invading source, the unwelcome toxins, and the body will heal!

It is very important to realize that people do not usually die as a result of a tumor. Rather, people die from the toxic burden a cancerous tumor causes.

Do not be frightened by the word cancer, as it is not the incurable mystery disease we have been led to believe. I experienced for myself that cancer can be defeated when the proper herbal remedies are taken and the body is detoxified.

This method of beating cancer is a very common-sense approach, and I followed three simple steps. The first step required eating the right foods, eliminating foods that feed the cancer-causing germs, as well as eliminating toxins, most especially chlorine and isopropyl alcohol, from my environment. Secondly, I destroyed the cancer-causing germs present in my body by using an herbal germ cleanse; and, finally, I removed the germs, bacteria, fungus and other toxins from my colon by using an enema or colonic.

Once I got well, I continue to maintain my good health by using 35% H202 on a daily basis.

Below is a list compiled by Dr. Clark explaining what food allergies she believed could trigger cancer.

Dr. Clark recommended that a person suffering with cancer avoid the foods which she found were related to different types of cancer.

ALLERGEN LOCATION TABLE

Cancer Location	Food Allergen (antigen)
abdominalmass (Onchocerca & lymph node)	CORN, SHRIMP
adrenal gland	mandelonitrile (almonds), *aldosterone*
Alveoli	D-mannitol (sugar variety)
Aorta	menadione (raw greens & grains)
Artery	hippuric acid (dairy products)
B- cells	*CORN, D-malic acid (malonic family)*
bile duct	acetic acid (vinegar)
Bladder	cinnamic acid
Bone	PIT, (cabbage)
bone marrow	limonene (lemon)
brain & spinal cord	caffeic acid (fruit, coffee)
Breast	apiol (soy products, oil)
Capillaries	*hippuric acid, pyrrole, benzoic acid*
cardiac (upper) stomach	phenol (derived from benzene)
Cartilage	Wheat
CD4's (T4 lymphocytes)	ASA (aspirin)
Cervix	ASA (aspirin)
chest mass (Dirofilaria & lymph node)	lactose (milk sugar),SHRIMP
choroid plexus (brain)	alphaketoglutaric acid
cochlea (ear)	cinnamic (cinnamon)
Colon	acetic acid, pyrrole, (blood, smoked food)
crista (ear)	malvin (red and blue fruits)
Diaphragm	NGF, (nerve growth factor), sardines, *mannitol*
epiglottis (throat)	naringenin (oranges), retinol (synthetic vitamin A)
Esophagus	menadione (synthetic Vitamin K)
esophagus, upper	menadione, *acetic acid, caffeic acid*
Eustachian tube	butter, beef

Eye	lily family (ONION, GARLIC, asparagus)
eye, iris	galacturonic acid (dairy products)
Fallopian tube	umbelliferone (carrots)
Fimbria	Chlorophyll
Gallbladder	acetic acid (vinegar)
Heart	tryptophane, tryptamine
heart (pacemaker, purkinje)	lactose (cow's milk)
Hodgkin's lymphoma	lactose, SHRIMP, *acetaldehyde*
Hypothalamus	chlorogenic acid
ileocaecal valve	*PIT (cabbage), naringenin (orange)*
Islets of Langerhans in . head region of pancreas . tail region of pancreas	quercetin (squash), phloridzin
Kidney	albumin, casein (dairy food, cheese)
ligamentum nuchae	limonene (citrus fruit)
Liver	umbelliferone (carrots)
lumbar spine	caffeic acid (caffeine)
Lung	coumarin (vanilla, rice, clover honey)
lung lymph nodes	L-tryptophan (milk)
lymph node	shrimp, (fish, seafood), *D-mannitol*
lymph vessel valve	Lactose
malignant melanoma	phenyl alanine plus mercury
medullated nerve	*apple* (not phloridzin), *caffeic acid* (caffeine)
medulla + 1 pF	dairy food, onion
Medulla	apiol, onion
medulla, left	tryptophane, piperine (black pepper) gallic acid (preservative in oil and grains)
megakaryocytes	aspirin, cinnamon
nipple and ducts of breast	dairy products, foods which contain aspartame
non-Hodgkin's lymphoma	shrimp & corn
nose, tip (nasal epithelium)	hippuric (food preservative) sodium pyruvate (red apple)

Omentum	limonene (citrus fruit)
osteomyelitis	Carrot
Ovary	dairy & oils
Pancreas	gallic acid (preservative in oil, grain)
Parathyroid	guanidine (not guanidine HCl) denaturant such as benzene
parotid gland (cheek)	hippuric acid (food preservatives)
Penis	ASA (aspirin)
peripheral nerve	apiol (oil), *caffeic acid*
pineal gland (brain)	*caffeic acid*
Pituitary	phloridzin (apple)
Platelets	limonene, D-malic acid
Prostate	acetic acid(vinegar), naringenin (orange)
RBC (red blood cells)	fructose (sugar in honey, corn syrup)
Rectum	NGF (nerve growth factor), D-mannitol
salivary glands	casein (dairy products)
seminal vesicle	ASA (aspirin)
skeletal muscle	melon (not cantaloupe), *lemon*
Skin	acetaldehyde, nuts, *NGF, apiol (oil)*
Sperm	glycine (amino acid)
spermatic cord	quercitin (squash)
Spleen	Peanut
stomach (all parts)	Phenol
sublingual gland	citric acid
submaxillary gland	eugenol (cloves)
Tendons	D-mannitol
Testis	phenylalanine (diet soda), D-tyramine (highest amounts found in aged cheeses & processed meats) glycine
Thymus	naringenin (orange)
Thyroid	D-tyramine, chlorine, fluorine, bromine
tongue, filiform	naringenin, MSG (monosodium glutamate), retinol, beta carotene
tongue, fungiform	ASA (aspirin), naringenin (orange), MSG, menadione (synthetic vitamin K), benzoic, retinol
Tonsil	ASA, naringenin, MSG, retinol, D- tyramine

Trachea	phenol (benzene), Phloridzin (apples)
Ureter	D-mannitol, avocado
Urethra	caffeic acid
Uterus	phenyl alanine (milk)
Vagina	acetaldehyde (chemical carcinogen), nuts, ASA(aspirin), *banana*
vas deferens	estrone (estrogenic)
Veins	menadione (synthetic Vitamin K)
vein valves	Corn

Food antigens invite the tumor nucleus to the allergic organ

(From "The Cure and Prevention of all Cancer", page 292-295; Copyright notice)

CHAPTER 10

How I Strengthened My Immune System

Come unto me, all ye that labor and are heavy laden,
and I will give you rest.—Matthew 11:28 KJV

When I developed cancer, I learned that one of the reasons I had the disease was my immune system was in a weakened state as the result of so many toxins in my body.

I learned that in order to get well, my immune system had to be strengthened. Chapter 18 provides an explanation of the importance Dr. Clark placed on the detox trio. The detox trio relieves the toxins in the immune system, allowing the white blood cells to do their work.

The next step I followed was an age-old and inexpensive technique I learned of from an old booklet Hannah loaned me; this booklet is no longer in print. The booklet was authored by Conrad LeBeau.

AN EASY METHOD TO STIMULATE AND STRENGTHEN THE IMMUNE SYSTEM

I purchased a bottle of cold pressed castor oil; the author cautions the castor oil must be cold pressed in order to be effective. I have made this product available on my website. As directed in the booklet, I massaged 2 tablespoons of castor oil into the right side of my lower abdomen, which is where 70% of the immune system is located. I then covered my lower right abdomen with BPA-free kitchen plastic wrap; I then placed a warm heating pad over the plastic wrap. The author advised that this be done daily and also said that doing this for 15 days will greatly strengthen the immune system. I tried making the time to do this twice a day for an hour each time. Rather than a heating pad, I used a far infrared hothouse, but a heating pad will work. A hothouse increases the effectiveness of the castor oil and makes using plastic wrap unnecessary. As with all of the equipment I mention, this type of hothouse is sold on my website. The hothouse is an awesome piece of equipment as it speeds the healing process.

I cut my finger severely with a food processor blade, leaving me with a wound that actually had 4 layers. It had the appearance of ground meat. I placed my hand in the hothouse that I had set on top of a far infrared sauna pad and covered it with a blanket. I tried to do this for hours at a time for 3 days. In 3 days my finger had healed. I have heard many testimonies of people who had wounds and broken bones and they too experience expedited healing. These are awesome items to have in the home.

The other area Conrad LeBeau recommend that a person focus on is the thymus gland, which is in the upper part of the chest, just below the neck; the author of the booklet recommends massaging the cold pressed castor oil over the area of the thymus, as well as tapping the thymus area with the middle and ring finger several times. The author's claim is that 2 tablespoons massaged and absorbed into the skin over these two areas daily will produce a stronger immune system in only a couple of weeks.

Mark Konlee has written a book entitled *How to Reverse Immune Dysfunction,* available on my website.

Failure to make any changes to our lifestyle following cancer surgery and just hoping for the best is lunacy.

A doctor might say, "Let's just keep our fingers crossed." However, we live in the information age today, and I think we all realize by now crossing our fingers isn't very effective! I learned there was something I could do to prevent cancer from taking my life!

I learned from Dr. Clark's book that in order to boost the immune system and enable the body to fight off illness, as the body was designed to, toxic products must be removed from the home environment.

Storing household cleaners and other items containing fragrance in the home is a serious matter. Manufactured fragrances suppress the body's ability to absorb oxygen into the cells, weakening the immune system and disrupting the hormones.

I learned the body stores toxins as we inhale them into the lungs, as well as accumulating them through direct contact with the body. The accumulation of these toxic substances eventually results in the dangerous condition known as estrogen dominance. As the result of estrogen dominance, the body begins to store fat and results in a weight gain that is nearly impossible to shed. With all of these toxins in our environment, it is easy to see why obesity has become a national epidemic here in the United States.

I learned that anyone desiring weight loss should first remove toxic items from their homes, as well as detoxifying their body by using a colon cleanse!

I found that non-organic commercial cleaning products adversely affect our endocrine system, as they act as hormone disruptors, linking them to the hormonal cancers, breast cancer and ovarian cancer. Just to make it clear, an endocrinologist specializes in the treatment of hormonal imbalances, which includes such problems as menopause, diabetes, metabolic disorders, lack of growth, osteoporosis, thyroid diseases, cancer of the endocrine glands, over-production or under-production of hormones, cholesterol disorders, hypertension and infertility.

So it was easy for me to understand why those nice-smelling fabric softeners were hazardous to my health, as are commercial room deodorizers, synthetic commercial perfumes, hygiene products with fragrance and fragrant candles!

Pesticides and herbicides, which contain xeno estrogens, have been formulated to attack an insect's reproductive system. I learned that these same pesticides also adversely affect our reproductive systems when we are exposed to them through the produce we eat or in our environment, wherever these toxins have been sprayed. Pesticide sprays are directly associated with estrogen dominance and hormonal cancer.

After discovering I had breast cancer, I discarded all of the fragrant products in my home and cancelled our monthly chemical lawn service. Our lawn was flawless. However, as I began to read Dr. Clark's book, *The Cure & Prevention of all Cancers*, I found there was a connection between breast cancer and xeno estrogens. When the company's home office inquired as to my reason for terminating the contract I had with them, I shared I was now suffering with breast cancer. The person on the other end of the line completely understood my decision.

Sadly, these estrogenic sprays make their way into our waterways and the entire ecosystem. Our beautiful wild birds and animals are drinking and wading through water polluted with these toxins; our fish are swimming in it. These lawns no longer even look appealing to me, but are really symbolic of the ignorance we have regarding the fragility of our precious ecosystem. What kind of legacy are we leaving to future generations? There are natural alternatives to pesticides and herbicides, and it would serve us all well to begin to seek out these solutions. You will find a wonderful book featured on my website, www.ibeatcancers.com, entitled *1001 All-Natural Secrets to Pest Control,* by Dr. Myles H. Bader.

I learned from reading a book by Dr. Cass Ingram that when a person has been exposed to pesticides, such as Agent Orange, they need to begin eating a lot of tomato sauce, preferably homemade tomato sauce, that contains no garlic or onions.

Another common source of hormone disruptors we can make almost daily contact with are cash register receipts, which are commonly coated with BPA resin. A good habit to make is to ask the cashier to place your register receipts into a plastic bag in order to avoid direct contact. According to an article I read on mercola.com, Dr. Mercola says it takes just two seconds for the hand to absorb BPA from the receipt. The state of Connecticut is the only state so far which has outlawed the use of BPA cash register paper.

Handling a lot of paperwork also exposes the body to dangerous estrogens as well and can also lead to estrogen dominance. Dry cleaned clothing is another source of hormone disrupting toxins introduced into the body.

I learned that eating cabbage, broccoli, or other cruciferous vegetables on a daily basis will help rid the body of harmful estrogens. DIM, DIM Plus or Women's Best Friend are all products which will pull harmful estrogens from the body.

Commercial anti-bacterial soaps and hand sanitizers must also be replaced, as they break down the immune system and disrupt hormonal balance. Replace them with essential oil formulas or formulate your own unique hygiene products by using organic essential oils. What an awesome gift for a loved one, your own homemade hand sanitizer made with essential oils, whether they are health-challenged or completely well!

I learned that in order to boost the immune system, probiotics should be part of the daily diet of everyone, and most especially for anyone who has a weakened immune system. In addition to the cabbage rejuvelac recipe featured in Chapter 32, sauerkraut and kimchi are two excellent sources of probiotics. I learned that turmeric, also called Curcumin, and vitamin D help to strengthen and rebuild the immune system.

Consumer Guide gave the brand Keybiotics the highest marks as a probiotic. My favorite brand of probiotics is Dr. Ohhira's Probiotics. They are packaged in a blister pack and travel easily. They are a bit pricey, but extremely effective in restoring gum health, as well as quickly repairing the colon. They can be purchased from my website, www.ibeatcancers.com. Hands down, Dr. Ohhira's Probiotics are to me the best available. According to the company, they can be taken 20 a day therapeutically, 10 in the a.m. and 10 in the p.m. This is an excellent way to re-establish good bacteria in the gut. I have heard testimonies of people who got sick while traveling, and they were able to fully recover very quickly by taking Dr. Ohhira's Probiotics in large doses.

Just a word of caution: The dairy industry recommends eating yogurt to supply the body with probiotics, and this is effective. However, if the dairy industry is plying its livestock with estrogens to insure a larger milk production, these harmful estrogens are then passed on to the consumer. Think organic dairy when choosing dairy as a healthy source of probiotics!

CHAPTER 11

Menopause & Alternative Solutions to HRT

We are troubled on every side, yet not distressed; we are perplexed, but not in despair, persecuted, but not forsaken; cast down, but not destroyed. – II Corinthians 4:8 & 9

The use of hormone replacement therapy, commonly referred to as HRT, is very often a choice made out of desperation. One of the symptoms of menopause, which contributes to the greatest amount of discomfort, hot flashes, is often lightheartedly referred to as personal summers. I can assure you though there is absolutely nothing amusing about a miserable condition which produces an overwhelming and debilitating sense of inner heat, followed by profuse sweating, and then ending with such a chill to the body that I need to crawl beneath a heavy winter blanket to get warm! This is distressing enough during the day, but when it occurs repeatedly at night, it serves to disrupt a good night's sleep. The following day the lack of sleep causes me to struggle with even the simplest activities. This pattern of sleep deprivation can go on for years.

However, Dr. Clark says using the detox trio mentioned in Chapter 18 will really help minimize hot flashes.

Some women sail through menopause and experience no difficulties. The chief complaint of many menopausal women is the inability to sleep or stay asleep.

When a woman suffers with sleep deprivation, she loses her mental acuity. Her thinking process often becomes foggy and dull, which serves to adversely affect every aspect of her life. Her emotions soon go unchecked, resulting in mood swings and rational thinking is out the window. The simple demands of life and relationships become overwhelming. The woman's physician may very often find it necessary to prescribe a pharmaceutical drug in order to help relieve anxiety.

So it is often out of desperation that a woman seeks hormone replacement therapy. There are many warnings associated with HRT, the most serious being cancer and heart disease. These warnings become a very distant secondary concern when the promise of life being somewhat restored to normal is dangled before the eyes of a woman in the throes of menopause.

Although HRT does indeed restore the joie de vivre, the French expression for the carefree joys of life, they do not come without a physical cost to the body. Unfortunately, when I made this desperate choice to seek relief using HRT, I had little realization of the toll it would take on my body.

Although I was familiar with the heightened dangers of developing cancer and heart disease relative to hormone replacement, I was unfamiliar with the fact I could actually counteract the side effects of HRT by adding some nutritional supplementation, and this lack of knowledge lent itself to the breakdown of my health.

Hormone replacement therapy upsets the delicate balance of life sustaining beneficial bacteria in the gut. According to Suzy Cohen, RPh, author of *Drug Muggers*, hormone replacement therapy also slowly drains the body of biotin, calcium, folate, magnesium, niacin, potassium, vitamin B6, riboflavin, selenium, thiamine, vitamin B12, vitamin C, vitamin D and zinc. These nutrients are absolutely vital in supporting a healthy immune system. So even though hormone replacement therapy offers relief from menopausal symptoms, its use weakens the immune system.

As a safe and effective alternative, I found that the use of Chinese Medicine can treat the symptoms of menopause without endangering health.

One of the products I learned of subsequent to my battle with cancer is Dr. Tagliaferri's Menopause Formula, which has no side effects. It is designed for women who want to avoid hormone therapy for fear of developing a hormonal cancer, heart disease, blood clots and stroke, all the side effects that come with hormone supplementation. This formula is based on Traditional Chinese Medicine's herbal remedies, used for thousands of years to treat menopausal symptoms. The plant-based ingredients in this proprietary product have been meticulously tested in clinical trials for safety and efficacy and are tested in the lab for batch-to-batch consistency.

Rather than supplementing with products which contain hormones, Traditional Chinese Medicine supplements the very essences from which the hormones are made. Traditional Chinese Medicine views menopause as the natural transition that leads a woman from the reproductive to the non-reproductive time in her life. At this age, hot flashes and night-sweats are caused in almost all cases by a root deficiency in the kidneys. It should be understood that diet and emotional stress have a strong impact on the intensity of hot flashes, and worry, anxiety, and fear can weaken and even damage the liver, which over time can deplete the kidneys even more, and increase the severity of the hot flashes. Junk foods, the wrong protein to carbohydrate balance, and too many sweets will elevate blood sugar levels, increase internal inflammation and add to the severity of the hot flashes and sweats. Incidentally, Dr. Hulda Clark spoke of a link between hot flashes and toxins in the kidneys.

The fundamental approach of Traditional Chinese Medicine at this stage of life is to boost and replenish the depleted kidney essence with natural substances that most closely resemble the ones in our bodies. The yin kidney essence is like the water in our automobile, controlling and balancing the fire from the engine. Herbal medicine is truly natural medicine and it is most effective for replenishing yin kidney essence.

Over the counter formulas based around Black Cohosh, Chaste Berries and Trifolium, create a mild estrogenic response in the body and even though they are effective in less severe instances of hot flashes, these herbs pose a dangerous threat to a cancer survivor.

More severe cases usually involve deep kidney yin deficiency with secondary imbalances in the liver and heart that can exacerbate anxiety and impair sleep. People will get best results from a yin rich formula that eliminates the fire by boosting the body's natural cooling waters.

Early oriental medical gynecologists discovered plants like Rehmannia, Anemarrhena and Phellodendron, whose molecular signatures nourish and replenish the deep essences of the kidneys. The patent formula, Zhi Bai Di Huang Wan (Anemarrhena and Phellodendron Combination) is safe and effective for most anyone suffering from hot flashes and overheating. Traditional Botanical Medicine's: "Great Essence Formula" combines ancient and modern wisdom for the treatment of hot flashes, overheating and the normal drying out of the body that occurs as we age, all without posing a threat to good health.

I learned to eat plenty of cruciferous vegetables on a regular basis, as this particular family of vegetables aids in ridding the body of harmful estrogens. Our bodies accumulate estrogen from HRT, as well as the harmful estrogens in the diet and the environment. There are products, such as DIM or DIM Plus or Women's Best Friend, which can aid in quickly flushing the body of harmful estrogens. These products are made from cruciferous vegetables.

In addition to supplementing with hormone replacement therapy, the toxins in our diets and our environments which lead to estrogen dominance are responsible for the near epidemic number of women who have developed hormonal cancers. I learned that removing the toxins that promote estrogen dominance was an absolute necessity if I wanted to fully recover from cancer! This meant eliminating the harmful estrogens from my diet and environment.

If I had the power to turn back the hands of time, I would not choose to use hormone replacement therapy. It is dangerous. I watched a very informative Canadian documentary entitled *"Our Daily Poison."* This documentary featured an interview with a French scientist who stated emphatically that supplementing with estrogen was always going to lead to the development of hormonal cancer.

If a woman uses HRT after having a bout with breast cancer, she must take it in conjunction with a chemotherapy drug, such as Tamoxifen. This type of drug requires close monitoring and is dispensed by an oncologist.

I purchased 100 percent bamboo sheets which also help me to sleep cooler, as bamboo sheets wick moisture away from the body, providing another avenue for some added relief. Sheets made from birch are also a good choice. I learned that regular exercise also served to greatly reduce hot flashes.

Many women in menopause suffer with vaginal dryness or vaginal atrophy, shrinking of the vagina, due to the loss of estrogen, and the use of Traditional Chinese Medicine, i.e., Dr. Mary Tagliaferri's formulas, address these symptoms beautifully. I wish I would have known about them when I went through menopause. Fennel oil is highly estrogenic oil and when applied directly onto the walls of the vagina, will prevent atrophy and the associated dryness that many women experience. This is a great alternative to estrogen creams. If a woman has suffered hormonal cancer, she must avoid fennel oil.

A few drops of myrtle oil blended with coconut oil and applied directly to the wall of the vagina will provide immediate relief for vaginal dryness, as well as greatly reduce the discomfort associated with the thinning of the vaginal walls due to the loss of estrogen. Myrtle oil is touted as being a natural product which enhances sexual pleasure. Clary sage oil is also used in treating vaginal dryness.

I learned taking pharmaceutical and over-the-counter drugs like ibuprofen or acetaminophen could seriously undermine my health, as drugs accumulate in the liver, eventually destroying a person's health. Rather than taking ibuprofen or acetaminophen for various aches and pains, I now take Phenocane made by OxyLife. Phenocane contains 250 mg. of Curcumin and also contains Nattokinase. Curcumin enhances the body's natural defense mechanism against inflammation and pain without harming the liver.

Curcumin is antifungal and has been found to be useful in the prevention of Alzheimer's disease. All disease is caused by inflammation, so taking a natural anti-inflammatory such as Curcumin would help prevent disease of any kind. Nattokinase aids in preventing blood clots.

Years ago, I sustained a herniated disc due to being rear-ended in a car collision, and I found that if I did too much strenuous activity during the day, I could experience throbbing pain at night, pain that kept me awake. I have discovered that the use of a far infrared pad for about 15 minutes will cause the pain to just melt away. The far infrared pad and several other amazingly useful pieces of equipment are featured in Chapter 45. These items are based upon Traditional Chinese Medicine and offer a healthy alternative to taking over-the-counter or pharmaceutical pain medication and offer many wonderful detoxifying properties, in addition to speeding the healing process. These wonderful products are available by going to www.ibeatcancers.com.

While I was going through the worst part of menopause, I suffered terribly with insomnia and experienced a couple of tangled encounters with sleeping pills; this is not an uncommon experience for a woman going through menopause.

Prescription sleeping medications come with serious side effects, but when you are desperate to get some sleep, it can seem like the only available option. Because of the insomnia that accompanies the condition of perimenopause and menopause, an addiction to prescription sleeping medication is not that unusual and can become a real nightmare to experience. I recall a massage therapist telling me that every middle-aged woman who worked in the doctor's office that employed her – and there were several middle-aged women working in the office—was addicted to the prescription drug Ambien, a popular pharmaceutical sleeping aid.

Once I started taking this medication, I started walking around my house in my sleep, according to family members, and once actually left the kitchen faucet running all night. Within 30 days of beginning the prescription, I felt really strung out, began to experience outbursts of anger and gained weight from eating in the middle of the night, one of the listed side effects. I actually woke up one night and realized I was eating out of a bowl of food in the refrigerator. I experienced the same problems the next time I tried a different brand of sleeping pills. I had to pray both times to break my addiction to sleeping pills, and I finally found a solution which provided me with a decent night's sleep: 2 to 3 capsules of L-Tryptophan by Lidtke, along with a cup of passion flower tea. I also read that supplementing with trace minerals would help resolve insomnia.

Urinary incontinence, frequency of urination or the sudden and urgent need to urinate can also be a problem for women who have reached menopause. I found the product SagaPro was an excellent remedy for this problem. Produced by EuroPharma, it is made with angelica herb leaf extract and promotes bladder strength and urinary tract function. My sleeping patterns improved because the number of times I had to rise during the night to urinate reduced to one and sometimes zero. SagaPro is also recommended for men and promotes prostate health.

Taking one of the many available 30 day herbal blend formulas which cleanse the kidneys and bladder also helped me to alleviate frequency of urination. I have a dear friend who has an adventurous spirit, and she and her husband, along with another couple, planned to hike a portion of the Appalachian Trail. She dreaded the thought of slowing her fellow hikers down by having to take too many "potty breaks." She purchased a kidney/bladder cleanse and was able to really enjoy her trip without the misery of constantly looking for a bush to hide behind!

Eliminating sugar and coffee from your diet can also decrease the severity of hot flashes during menopause. Unless you make the decision to stop drinking coffee and other caffeinated beverages, you may not stop experiencing the difficult symptoms of menopause. Coffee drains the adrenal glands, and the adrenal glands must be functioning properly in order to regulate the ideal amount of estrogen in the body. Once the ovaries stop producing estrogen, the adrenals take over. So maintaining healthy adrenal glands can mean aging gracefully, good health and a great sex life, as well. Life is full of choices, and this is another choice we get to make.

The biggest struggle I had during this entire menopausal ordeal was to stop drinking coffee. Oh, how I love coffee! I love the chatty buzz, which coincidentally annoys my husband to no end.

Chaga is a great coffee substitute, and it also reportedly serves to protect the body from cancer. Chaga is a medicinal mushroom or fungus which grows on birch trees and is recognized in Russia and Europe as containing healing properties. It is an excellent product to use to build and strengthen the immune system. It contains SOD, super oxide dismutase, which slows the aging process. According to Dr. Cass Ingram, the North American Indians of Canada used chaga as a curative for cancer. Chaga makes you strong! Chaga is sold by the North American Herb & Spice Company and is marketed in several ways: A selection including Chaga drops; Chaga syrup; Chaga White; my favorite, Chaga Black; Chaga Chunks, yummy; among other products, are available on my website, www.ibeatcancers.com.

Dr. Ingram advises that chaga is an excellent way to rebuild strength for someone who is in a weakened state. The North American Herb & Spice Company does recommend that you NOT USE CHAGA WHILE TAKING ANTIBIOTICS OR CHEMOTHERAPY!

As I entered menopause, my fingernails weakened, and I experienced vertical ridges and splitting down the middle of my fingernails, which was quite painful. A couple of months after I began drinking a cup of chaga every day, I discovered my fingernails had become much stronger and no longer split. I no longer had to resort to wearing toxic products, like artificial nails, nail polish and glue to keep my fingernails intact. When I began supplementing with 35% H202, my nails became even stronger.

As I mentioned in the chapter already, Dr. Clark wrote that there are other sources of hot flashes besides hormonal imbalance. She said that you can also experience hot flashes when your white blood cells are unable to release toxins into the kidneys, allowing for the toxins in the body to be flushed through the kidneys and released into the bladder. She recommended taking the detox trio described in Chapter 18, wild source Vitamin C, hydrangea root and selenium, which she said will bring relief from this type of hot flashes.

Another very common reason to experience hot flashes, particularly at night, according to Dr. Clark, is the cancer-causing germ overload in the body. Dr. Clark said taking her herbal germ cleanse, which appears in Chapter 19, will bring quick relief from this type of hot flashes.

Eventually, I learned the therapeutic use of 35% H202 would be effective in eliminating this type of hot flashes for only pennies a day. Read about my experience in Chapter 22.

CHAPTER 12

Chlorine & Our Immune System

*And they shall teach my people the difference between
the holy and the common, and cause them to discern
between the unclean and the clean.*—Ezekiel 44:23 KJV

I learned if there is a desire to live long and strong, eliminating exposure to chlorine is mandatory. Chlorine damages our health because it breaks down the immune system by killing the healthy bacteria in the gut. Without a healthy immune system, the body is susceptible to sickness and unable to recover from disease. Envision a rock being thrown through a plate glass window; the result will be the window is shattered; this is what chlorine does to your immune system. Chlorine breaks down metal and plastic; imagine what its effect must be on your body!

Dr. Hulda Clark wrote in her book, *The Cure & Prevention of all Cancers*, that it is impossible to recover from cancer while chlorine is present in the environment. She warns chlorine is a known carcinogen which prevents the immune system from defending the body against disease. Chlorine is a causative factor in all hormonal cancers as it promotes estrogen dominance.

However, Dr. Clark recommended the use of NSF-certified bleach as a safe alternative. NSF-certified bleach can be purchased at a pool supply store. My grocery store carries it. Dr. Clark reported it is safer to clean and do laundry with this type of bleach. You will want to protect against direct skin contact with NSF-certified bleach, but she said it does not pose the same threat to your health as does regular chlorine bleach.

City water departments are required to use NSF-certified bleach to treat the tap water for its citizens, rather than what we know as ordinary household chlorine bleach.

According to Dr. Clark, city water treated with household laundry bleach can be heavily contaminated with azo dyes, PCB's, benzene, asbestos and heavy metals, all of which are substances associated with the disease of cancer. If you have good, clean well water at your disposal, rather than chlorinated city water, you are truly blessed indeed! Drinking chlorinated water as a child will result in poor kidney function as an adult.

Products marketed as immune system builders are limited in their abilities, as they can only enhance white blood cell function. These products cannot replace the function of white blood cells. To fully recover from disease, the white blood cells of the immune system must be able to perform their function. The white blood cells are weakened and disabled when chlorine is present. Our ability to have access to pure, chlorine-free drinking water and our ability to bathe in water free of chlorine are absolutely crucial to good health.

Chlorine does serve to protect our water supply, but once it reaches our home, we must protect ourselves from chlorine. Today when chlorine is used to purify community water, it is most likely a substance called chloramine, which is a mixture of chlorine and ammonia, with other additives being fluoride and bromine, two other chemical agents which are also very harmful to health and are associated with estrogen dominance. Dr. Clark said it is possible to keep the cancer at bay while using water treated with chlorine, but, in her opinion, the cancer will not be cured while chlorine is present.

According to the late Dr. Linus Pauling, the substances in chlorinated water create electronegativity. Simply put, these chemicals displace the presence of iodine in the body, weakening the thyroid and thus weakening the body. In addition, these chemicals added to our water supply disrupt the body's mitochondrial process by robbing the cells of oxygen. The mitochondria are known as the powerhouse of the cell; the mitochondria charge the body with energy. The end result of continual exposure to chlorine, ammonia, bromine, and fluoride will be a reduction in the body's energy! As chlorine displaces iodine in the body, thyroid problems will surface, leading to obesity and hair loss. I learned I could combat the harmful effects of these toxins by oxygenating my body using distilled water and a few drops 35% food grade hydrogen peroxide, which would greatly aid in rebuilding my immune system. I explain my experience in Chapter 22. This can be done for just pennies a day.

You can purchase a range of water distillers, as well as purchasing chlorine filtering showerheads and systems by going to www.ibeatcancers.com.

According to Dr. Clark, the supplement MSM breaks up the cancer-causing complex created by chlorine and should therefore be a supplement included in the daily regimen of those who use city water, swim in a chlorinated pool or make use of a Jacuzzi treated with a chlorine product.

Rather than using any type of bleach as a cleaning agent in the home, with the exception of sterilizing your sinks and toilet with NSF bleach, choose essential oils as an alternative to using cleaning products which contain harmful ingredients.

The chapter entitled "Simplicity of Life" lists many essential oils and how they can be used in the home. You can purchase products formulated with essential oils to use as safe and effective cleaning agents or you can formulate your own essential oil cleaning products.

Rather than breaking down your health cleaning with products which contain harmful toxins, these wonderful essential oils will kill germs and bacteria, and, at the same time, help build and strengthen your immune system!

CHAPTER 13

Harmful Dyes

A woman named Lydia ... sold purple
dye for a living.—Acts 16:14

Unlike in times of old when the source of dyes was derived naturally, the
dyes utilized in products we use today are typically created in a laboratory
and are very often dangerous substances that pose a real threat to good
health. Yellow, red, and blue food dyes contain harmful neurotoxins that
have an adverse effect on the brain. These food dyes are most frequently
found in bakery items, such as decorated cakes, cookies, candies and
similar desserts, but their use is not confined to the bakery, as they are also
commonly found in many processed foods and beverages.

Consumption of these dyes can dramatically affect a child's behavior,
and the dangerous neurotoxins remain in the brain tissue long after the
party is over. Children are not the only ones to be adversely affected by
these dyes; the elderly and infirm are also especially vulnerable to these
toxic substances, and researchers warn that food dyes can have a dangerous
interaction with prescription drug medications, as well.

To enhance the appearance of raw beef, a well-known bargain
supermarket uses red dye. Because dyes are ingredients in so many foods
and beverages, we must read labels to protect our health. Some dyes may
not even appear on the package because they are considered an industry
standard. The accumulation of these chemical additives consumed in our
diets can add up to something sizable enough to become a menace to our
good health. As well as being associated with cancer, food dyes are also

linked to asthma, autism, ADHD, anxiety, depression, as well as many other diseases.

Another dangerous substance in the marketplace we can be exposed to today is azo dye, also called phenylenediamine. Dr. Clark alleged in her books that the dye used on beef in bargain supermarkets is phenylenediamine. I do not know if this is still true today. However, phenylenediamine is currently used in commercial hair dye. At one time, phenylenediamine was used in margarine to give it a deep yellow color. The use of this dye in all foods was outlawed in the United States in the 1940s, as it was found to be carcinogenic, but its presence slipped past legislators as an ingredient in hair dye. Dr. Clark claimed traces of phenylenediamine or azo dye as it is commonly known was present in every breast tumor she personally dissected and analyzed. It is an established fact that hair dye containing this substance is a principal cause of lymphoma.

Purchase an azo dye-free hair color from www.ibeatcancers.com, and ask your hairdresser to kindly accommodate your desire to change products or find a hairdresser who uses organic hair products. Hairdressers who use exclusively organic products are growing in numbers, as they themselves and their savvy customers have learned of the connection which exists between disease and the chemicals so often used in beauty and hygiene products.

In an online Alternative News Health Letter, I was able to gather some very sobering facts. I read phenylenediamine was claimed to be responsible for the increased risk of non-Hodgkin's lymphoma, as well as other cancers. Phenylenediamine, which is often preceded by the letter m, o, or p, in labeling is usually found in permanent dyes commonly known as oxidation dyes or peroxide dyes. Protected under the 1938 FDA exemption which Dr. Clark alluded to, this particular chemical has been shown to cause cancer in animal experiments, and at least two studies have shown that repeated exposure to phenylenediamine increases the risk of bladder cancer in humans. A recent study conducted by researchers at the University of Southern California found that women who routinely dye their hair are more than three times as likely to develop bladder cancer. Another study of more than 45,000 hairdressers by researchers at Sweden's Karolinska Institute found that frequent exposure to the chemicals in hair dye also increases the risk of lung, colon and upper digestive cancers.

Although the FDA is unable to ban its use due to the exemption, the agency proposed a requirement ordering manufacturers to place warning labels on products containing this substance. If the proposal had been accepted, the label would have read, "Warning: [this product] contains an ingredient that can penetrate your skin and has been determined to cause cancer in laboratory animals." At the same time, the FDA also proposed that beauty salons using these products post warnings for their customers. As it happens, however, the powerful cosmetic industry wasn't going to take this lying down; and their lobbyists successfully defeated both proposals; so no warnings were ever placed on the products containing this dangerous chemical.

Phenylenediamine isn't the only hazardous substance found in hair dyes. Coal tar colors, which are listed on hair dye labels as FD&C or D&C colors, are derived from the tar found in bituminous coal. Dr. Cass Ingram stated that coal tar is the single most toxic, cancer-causing substance on the planet. Coal tar contains benzene, a substance which was banned from a number of household products in the 1970's because it increases the risk of leukemia. What this means is there was such a sudden increase in leukemia cases that alarmed researchers quickly tried to put an end to the use of benzene.

Some coal tar also contains heavy metal impurities, including lead and arsenic, both of which cause cancer and can disrupt hormones. Although many of the synthetic colors used in hair dyes have never been tested for safety, the World Health Organization considers them all possible carcinogens.

A study by Xavier University in New Orleans found that the gradual hair dyes many men use contained so much lead acetate that the researchers couldn't wash it off of their hands. Based on this and studies that were similar in nature, the Center for Environmental Health, a San Francisco-based non-profit group, sued Combe, Inc., the makers of Grecian Formula, for violation of California's Proposition 65. Although the suit was settled and Combe reformulated the hair dyes to reduce the amount of lead acetate, lead is a cumulative chemical and even low levels of exposure can ultimately result in cancer, brain damage, muscle weakness and depression.

Check out the selection of organic hair dye on my website! Also, check out the great selection of non-toxic beauty products, at www. ibeatcancers.com.

CHAPTER 14

The Hazards of Ultra-pasteurized and Non-organic Dairy

As newborn babes, desire the sincere milk of the word
that you may grow thereby.—1 Peter 2:2 KJV

When a milk container reads "ultra-pasteurized" milk, this means it has been sterilized by forcing the milk through superheated metal plates which contain cobalt. This method of processing milk has been adopted by the dairy industry in order to increase the shelf life of fresh milk for up to three months; according to an article I read which was published by the prestigious Weston A. Price Foundation.

The creator of "ultra-pasteurized" milk was an Italian company which pitched their methods of shelf life extension to the dairy industry in the United States. They were indeed able to hit the nail on the head as far as increasing the shelf life of milk, as ultra-pasteurized milk can be left on the kitchen counter for weeks, and it will not sour.

The process of ultra-pasteurizing flattens the protein molecules in milk making the enzymes in milk no longer beneficial, but instead become hazardous to our health. Ingesting ultra-pasteurized dairy products causes a condition in the colon called leaky gut. When the flattened protein molecules pass into the bloodstream through a leaky gut, the body perceives them as foreign proteins and mounts an immune response. This results in a chronically overstressed immune system and much less energy available for growth and repair. People feed this milk to their children thinking it is a nutritious beverage. It isn't! Ultra-pasteurized dairy products pose a serious threat to good health and should be completely avoided.

As the result of the ultra-pasteurizing process, the milk takes on a cabbage-like flavor and then becomes stale, bitter, and gelatinous—and this all happens before it is shipped off to the store. The writer of the Weston A. Price Foundation article, together with other investigators, surmises that some kind of flavorings or other chemicals are added to the milk in order to combat this problem. If the whole industry does this, they are not required to list such additives because it is considered an "industry standard." This milk is dead and cannot even be used to make yogurt, as it will not set up.

Concerned scientists assert that there are foreign compounds in the ultra-pasteurized milk as the result of heating and storage, and these compounds accumulate in the body, producing negative effects on the endocrine system. The glands in the endocrine system secrete hormones within the body. These hormones influence such things as metabolic activity (the breakdown of ingested food into energy), reproduction, mood, growth, and body development. Consequently, consuming ultra-pasteurized milk is considered a way to introduce substances which disrupt hormones in the body. Obviously, this milk has little to offer in the way of nutritional value.

Request that your grocer provide pasteurized milk rather than ultra-pasteurized.

Choosing organic dairy which is not ultra-pasteurized is not the only concern you should have when selecting dairy products. The dairy industry has another dangerous money-making method used to increase their profits. To ensure maximum milk production, many farmers now routinely inject dairy cattle with cancer-causing synthetic hormones, rBGH and rBST. The use of these hormones on dairy cattle is outlawed in the European Union, Australia, Canada, Israel, and New Zealand. These nations will not purchase our dairy products neither will they buy our meats. They are sending the American consumer a frightening message!

One simply will not get well or remain cancer-free if ingesting these non-organic dairy products. Even if a woman is not suffering with cancer, she would do well to avoid non-organic dairy, as the high estrogen levels in these products will wreak havoc with her menstrual cycle by causing estrogen dominance. Non-organic dairy products will put a woman, any woman, regardless of her age at an increased risk of developing hormonal cancer.

I spoke to a woman in her 70's who shared with me she had begun to suffer once again with hot flashes. She had gone through menopause 20 years earlier, and suddenly she felt as though she was beginning menopause all over again. She was completely mystified by these symptoms. I asked if she had been consuming a lot of dairy products lately.

"Yes. I've been eating a lot of cheese," she responded, giving me a very surprised expression. I then inquired as to whether the cheese she was eating was organic. She responded that it was not. I explained to her that she was ingesting large enough amounts of estrogen to generate hot flashes. This was her body's way of warning her if she didn't switch to organic cheese, she could very well develop a hormonal cancer.

The dairy industry is in business to make money, and no one can or should fault them for this. However, when the dairy industry takes measures to increase their milk production at the expense of the consumer's health, and government agencies do not step in to protect the consumer, the consumer must make informed choices in order to protect their own health. Any dairy farmers who are employing these methods are gradually destroying their customers' health. Unless changes are made to cease from these unscrupulous business practices, they will prove to be the downfall of the industry.

This type of animal husbandry is nothing short of insanity and is a dark and shameful side of the dairy industry. Just as humans develop hormonal cancers as a result of estrogen supplementation, cattle are also sickened by hormonal cancers and sent to the slaughterhouse for their next appearance as fast food burgers. This means fast food beef burgers can contain extremely high levels of estrogen.

Organic dairy products do provide much beneficial nutrition and calories for those suffering with cancer. However, according to Dr. Clark, some cancers, such as certain brain cancers and breast cancers are actually triggered by the body's allergic reaction to dairy. I have learned this: If you do not care for dairy products or are lactose intolerant, this may be a good sign that dairy does not agree with your body type, meaning that it is possibly an allergen for you and should be avoided. Some people may experience constipation as the result of eating dairy products. Dr. Clark recommended taking frequent but small doses of wild source vitamin C throughout the day in order to keep the bowels gently moving.

Dr. Clark said the consumption of raw milk is preferable, as it contains a special factor called lactoferrin. This factor is missing from the liver, spleen, and bone marrow of anemia and cancer patients. One glass of raw milk will replenish this essential factor for over a week. Raw milk is often marketed as milk for pets in order to avoid strict regulations placed on raw dairy distributors by the federal government. You should be able to locate a dairy near you by going to RealMilk.com.

If raw dairy products are unavailable to you, use the available pasteurized products, making sure that you purchase only products which have labels that assure no antibiotics or hormones were used to treat their dairy cattle.

Regardless of whether the dairy products are raw or pasteurized, Dr. Clark stressed it is extremely important to sterilize dairy before consumption. The effort must be made to follow through with the sterilization process of milk, cream, cheese and butter in order to destroy the many germs and bacteria which the weakened immune system is simply unable to manage.

I included Dr. Clark's directions for sterilizing milk in Chapter 32, but I subsequently learned that a few of drops of 35% food grade hydrogen peroxide would sterilize an 8 ounce glass of milk.

Dr. Clark said it is unnecessary to sterilize dairy products which are heated in cooking. Organic cheese or ozonated cheese may be eaten without sterilization if they are baked. Avoid Gorgonzola and blue cheeses; although these cheeses have a unique and delicious taste, they contain a high amount of fungus. I often enjoy a delicious commercial cheese made with almond milk.

I learned that organic dairy products have a significantly important place in our daily diets. They are actually medicinal. Aside from the much-touted probiotics, organic dairy aids in healing and strengthening the body. Organic milk contains CLA, conjugated linoleic acid, a substance that protects the body against free radicals that lead to cancer development. Organic cottage cheese, along with sacha inchi oil or good quality flaxseed oil, will heal bladder cancer, according to the late Dr. Johanna Budwig, one of Germany's top biochemists, who promoted natural alternative cancer solutions. Years ago I met a gentleman who was a paraplegic and had been plagued with constant bladder infections. He shared with me that he was constantly taking antibiotics until he learned that he could prevent these bladder infections by eating a small serving of organic cottage cheese with a tablespoon of flax seed oil two or three times a day.

The most important thing I learned is that dairy must be sterilized or treated with 35% H202 before it is consumed by a person suffering with cancer.

CHAPTER 15

Environmental Toxins

> My people are destroyed for lack of
> knowledge.—Hosea 4:6 KJV

Previous to the revelation that there was a connection between my breast tumor and exposure to toxins and metals, I was not a label reader at all. I happily went along in life, completely uninformed. I was far too busy to be bothered by any information about what might pose a threat to my health. I had places to go and appointments to keep because I was taking care of myself—either my weekly visits to the hairdresser, the massage therapist, the spa for a facial, or my bi-weekly visits to the nail spa for a manicure and pedicure. Unbeknownst to me, I was constantly being exposed to products which were detrimental to my health. I even realized my gym was another place I was encountering toxic cleaning products.

It wasn't until I found out the tumor in my breast would not completely dissolve unless I eliminated my exposure to products which contained toxic substances, primarily the solvent isopropyl alcohol as well as chlorine that I sat up and paid attention.

I learned the typical breast tumor contains solvents, toxins, and metals; substances I was exposed to on a daily basis in my own home. I also learned I would never fully recover from cancer if I didn't do something about eliminating these substances from my environment. If I was going to recover my health, I alone had the responsibility of carefully examining the labeled ingredients of every product I planned on applying to my skin, and I alone had the responsibility of removing toxic cleaning products and replacing them with items that did no harm to my immune system. I alone was responsible for eliminating estrogen dominance in my body.

I had been cornered by cancer and forced into taking a proactive approach in order to keep all of my body parts intact and survive this disease! I was shocked to learn I had singlehandedly built my own tumor!

The first startling revelation I received from reading Dr. Hulda Clark's book, *The Cure & Prevention of all Cancers,* was the sinister role isopropyl alcohol played in malignancy. I learned from her book I would not remain cancer free if I did not discontinue the use of this dangerous solvent, which was an ingredient in everything I was applying to my skin, including perfume. Isopropyl alcohol is also called isopropanol, glycol or a variety of other names that include the letters P-R-O-P.

I learned commercial laundry detergent was actually made from petroleum, rather than soap, and that petroleum based laundry detergent was introducing dangerous toxins into my body. Go to www.ibeatcancers.com to find a vast selection of available laundry products that are toxin free.

See Chapter 27 for more information on non-toxic laundry and cleaning alternatives which are affordable.

The beauty of the far infrared sauna and the ion foot cleanse is these two pieces of detoxification equipment are extremely useful in removing toxins from the body. Unless we utilize some measure of detoxifying our body on a regular basis, we will continue to store toxins.

We also accumulate and store metals, which promotes the growth of fungus in the body. We collect metal from copper water pipes, pollution and chlorinated water. Fungus is the very foundation of a tumor.

The presence of copper in the bloodstream will foster a continual fungal infection in the body and can prevent a cancerous tumor from completely dissolving. Most likely, all of us have seen what happens to a copper penny when it is left in a moist, warm spot. The penny turns a fungus green. This is exactly what happens when copper sits in the body.

According to Dr. Clark, all cancerous tumors contain inorganic copper, and cancer researchers have known for years there is a correlation between inorganic copper and cancer. When I began to research the connection between cancer and copper on the Internet, I was astounded by the number of articles linking the disease of cancer with inorganic copper. Aside from it being linked to cancer, inorganic copper in the body is associated with high blood pressure, hair loss, and weight gain, among many other health issues.

Copper is also found in jewelry, dental metal, and cookware. If you suffer with cancer and live in an older home that has copper water pipes, Dr. Clark advised that you need to make a change or your tumor will not completely dissolve. She warned that you will be more susceptible to fungal infection in your body when your home is equipped with copper piping.

According to Dr. Clark, unless copper is completely eliminated from your drinking water and the water you bathe in, there cannot be a full recovery from cancer. Cancer will go into remission as the result of the herbal remedy, but it will not be fully healed until exposure to copper is eliminated.

As long as one lives in a home equipped with copper water piping, the body is exposed to copper and will continue to collect more copper. Estrogen has the dangerous effect of actually pulling copper into the body and holding it there, not allowing copper residue to enter the bladder and be released into the urine.

There is a coating marketed which is blown into copper pipes to prevent the copper from seeping into water. This is referred to as CIPP—cured in place piping.

Copper is by no means the only metal that poses a threat to health. Aluminum is another metal to avoid. As convenient as it may be to use aluminum foil in the kitchen, when there is a problem with the immune system, it should be avoided. Drinking beverages from aluminum cans should be absolutely avoided.

Aluminum is used to line the inside of many products packaged in soft packaging. Among those products are juice boxes and juice packs, products marketed directly toward the very young. I learned the aluminum in this lining attacks the kidneys, and that this exposure to aluminum has the ability to take down a child's kidneys very quickly. Although this packaging may be very convenient, this is not healthy packaging and should be avoided.

I learned the metals that pose the greatest threat to your health are the ones placed there by your dentist. I attended a health seminar on the subject of alternative medicine while gathering information for this book.

The very first words out of the mouth of the guest speaker when he stood up were, "There is an old saying: 'If we did not have dentists, we would not need doctors.'" The speaker went on to explain the danger metal dental work poses to the body.

If you follow the prescribed approach Dr. Clark recommended—using the powerful herbal remedies, completely avoiding the foods that encourage the presence of cancer-causing germs, avoiding moldy foods or foods that mold easily, avoiding isopropyl alcohol, as well as eliminating your exposure to other toxins—and the tumor has perhaps reduced in size, but is not completely gone, your metal dental work may be preventing the complete restoration of your health. Consistent detoxing can effectively remove these metals from the bloodstream.

Dr. Clark asserts that mercury amalgam fillings, as well as other dental metals, are a burden to the immune system and even the noble metals, gold and silver are very toxic to the body! She advises the removal of these metals. I did not follow this advice, but I do make a habit of detoxing.

You may very likely find that your dentist may be upset by this assertion and will heatedly dispute this information, dismissing it as being totally without merit and nonsensical, as it is a very controversial subject. The claim dental metals are toxic to the body is a widespread assertion among the alternative medicine community and makes perfect sense. Contrariwise, the argument of the American Dental Association is simply vehement denial.

If a person makes the decision to follow Dr. Clark's advice, there are dentists who specialize in the removal of metal in the mouth, and they are fully informed about the dangers these metals pose to your health. This is who you want for the job—a specialist, a dentist who has been specifically trained to do the job of metal removal. This is your life we're talking about here! Take care to choose wisely when making your selection of a dentist; do some research. It would be best to locate a dentist through the recommendation of the International Academy of Oral Medicine and Toxicology (IAOMT); this agency will provide a list of qualified dentists worldwide.

Find out as much as possible about the dentist's methods. Ask if they provide the patient with an alternative source of air during the removal process, if they employ a rubber dam, and whether they use air abrasion technology for final cleanup of amalgam and plastic. These three processes are important to insure safe removal. In my opinion, it would be preferable if the dentist came highly recommended by another patient who previously had dental metals removed. An independently owned health food store may be a good source when seeking information recommending a qualified dentist.

If my health was challenged and I made a decision to have the dental metals removed, this is what I would do: I would make sure I began to eat plenty of fiber and begin taking an herbal preparation which removes metals from the body. These are available at a good health food store. I would also plan to have a few colonic hydrotherapy procedures in order to get things moving along. These are all very important measures to aid in removing any heavy metals which have seeped into the body.

I would also employ the use of a far infrared sauna or an ion cleanse foot detox during this time, to clean up any metals which may have seeped into my bloodstream. These two items of equipment are recommended as providing for optimum results in the quest to rid the body of heavy metals. The sauna is most effective when the temperature is around 100 degrees, which will produce a gentle sweat. Higher temperatures may actually serve to drive the metals deeper into the body.

I read that for optimum results fourteen ion cleanse foot detox procedures should be taken two or three days apart within a two-month period to remove metals from the body, and then to follow up with a weekly foot detox. In my experience with the foot detox, I saw small metal shards at the bottom of the foot detox water. I learned it is imperative to drink plenty of water during the sauna or foot cleanse. Far infrared saunas of varying prices, as well as an ion cleanse foot detox, are available at www.ibeatcancers.com.

A gentleman who owns a company which manufacturers an ion cleanse foot detox claims he was healed of lung cancer using this detoxification tool. He was so impressed by the effectiveness of the foot detox that he purchased the company.

As popular as they may be, dental implants are extremely dangerous, according to Dr. Clark, because a metal post is implanted into the gum. What this translates to for the individual is toxic metal is actually plugged directly into the immune system. She claimed that this procedure has the potential of being exceedingly harmful to one's good health.

After reading about the dangers of these dental metals and the problems associated with them, I happened to meet a seventy-eight-year-old woman who suffered with a tumor in her mouth. The tumor, which had quickly developed, was as big around as a large marble. The woman told me she was no longer able to chew and took all of her nourishment in liquid form. She sought help through her dentist, who advised her to consult with her physician. I related my experience with the Juice of Wild Oreganol, as well as the benefits I experienced with the herbal germ cleanse.

I mentioned to this lady that I had learned that the tumor might very possibly be the result of dental metal, and she most likely had cancer in her lymphatic system as well. She then told me the tumor was growing right alongside a metal crown and she, herself, had wondered whether there was a connection between the metal crown and the tumor. The woman told me she had requested the dentist pull the tooth, but he did not want to work near the tumor and refused to do an extraction.

I shared with her how I sterilized dairy products and washed produce, explaining the importance of avoiding re-infection of dangerous germs and bacteria while she battled disease. I also shared with her about the dangers of isopropyl alcohol and the necessity of avoiding toxins, primarily chlorine.

She later related to me she had purchased the Juice of Wild Oreganol and an herbal cleanse and then informed me by e-mail a few days later her tumor had shrunk considerably, enabling her to chew soft foods. Rather than giving the natural treatment any more time, she planned on keeping a scheduled appointment she had with a prestigious cancer treatment center in Tampa as the result of a referral she received from her physician. She had a daughter who lived out of state who was insisting her mother see a cancer specialist. I knew the culmination of her appointment would be hospitalization and her hospitalization would include exposure to isopropyl alcohol, which would serve to quickly create a setback in her health, but I said nothing to discourage her decision.

I later learned through her husband things did not go well at the cancer treatment center. She was subjected to extensive surgery, as they did indeed locate cancer in her lymphatic glands, and her health rapidly deteriorated while she was hospitalized. She deeply regretted not following through with natural medicine. Her husband informed me that she started taking the Juice of Wild Oreganol as soon as she was released from the hospital.

Some months later, I heard what this poor lady endured during hospitalization. Part of her tongue was removed, a lot of her gums, as well as many lymph nodes. She was now committed to pursuing good health using alternative methods. I felt sorry to hear she had lost part of her tongue, her gums and lymph nodes, as the lymphatic system powerfully battles disease for the body. The removal of lymph nodes creates a lifelong problem with swelling.

The lymphatic system can be compared to a sewer system in the body which collects toxic waste from the bloodstream. I learned from reading books by Dr. Cass Ingram that the lymphatic system can be easily cleansed by taking the Juice of Wild Oreganol.

Around this same time a lady who was in her 60's and had been diagnosed with untreatable stage 4 lung cancer, which had metastasized to other organs, contacted me. She followed through with both of the herbal cleanses, the Juice of Wild Oreganol, as well as the herbal combination of black walnut, wormwood and cloves, and she was vastly improved, but got very little relief with her labored breathing. It was at this point I asked her if she had gold fillings. Yes, she responded, declaring her mouth had nothing but gold fillings and crowns. She was very proud of this fact.

I explained to her what I had read in Dr. Clark's book regarding gold in the teeth. Dr. Clark's book, The Cure and Prevention of all Cancers, states the presence of gold within the body produces prions, and these prions prevent the healing of--most specifically--lung cancer.

Dr. Clark recommends using a mixture of 35% food grade hydrogen peroxide and distilled water as a mist, spraying on the back of the throat several times a day, for the treatment of lung cancer. She stressed that when gold is present in the teeth nothing will cure lung cancer. She stated this does not necessarily mean you will succumb to the lung cancer, but it does mean as long as the gold is present you will battle the lung cancer. Directions for the hydrogen peroxide solution that Dr. Clark recommended can be located on the Internet in a simple search, i.e., Lung Cancer, Hydrogen Peroxide and the genius of Hulda Clark.

After researching this information, I learned of a book called *Hydrogen Peroxide, Medical Miracle,* by Dr. William Campbell Douglass. I explained my wonderful experience with 35% food grade hydrogen peroxide in Chapter 22.

The lady suffering with lung cancer strongly disagreed with Dr. Clark's advice concerning removal of gold dental work. I was able to give her food for thought in our last conversation though. The lady professed to be a Bible-believing Christian, so I mentioned to her a passage in Exodus 32. Moses forced the Israelites to drink water mixed with gold dust as a punitive measure after they financed the creation of a golden calf by donating their earrings. When Moses arrived on the scene after spending 40 days at the top of a mountain with God and saw the people worshiping the golden calf, he really lost his cool. He burned the idol, ground it to powder, and mixed it with water that descended from the mountain of God. The people who were forced to drink this noxious elixir all died at 70 years of age.

Doesn't it seem more than just a bit odd that all who were forced to drink this heavy metal cocktail died at exactly 70 years of age?

The ADA alleges dental metal poses no threat to health. I believe there is definitely credence to Dr. Clark's claim of these metals being hazardous to one's health. After reading several Internet articles and health books which describe the toxicity associated with dental metal and the threat they pose to good health, along with viewing the 60 Minutes segment entitled "Is There Poison In Your Mouth" on Youtube, it is easy to grasp the validity of Dr. Clark's admonition.

Removing these metals from the mouth may seem like a drastic move; however, if you are unable to recover your health in any other way, it is well worth the consideration of having the metals removed. Many who practice daily detoxing say it is possible to eliminate the threat of these metals to your health when you make detoxification a daily habit. I have a friend who has many mercury amalgam fillings, but detoxes faithfully every day. She shared with me that a recent blood draw tested negative for the presence of mercury.

There are dentists in Mexico who specialize in this type of metal removal and replacement with an acceptable product. Choosing a dentist from Mexico for metal removal could very well prove to be a cost-saving choice, excluding transportation and lodging, of course. However, a friend of mine who chose to go to one of these Mexican dental clinics to have her dental metal removed told me she was disappointed with the results. She visited a dentist in her local area specializing in metal removal once she returned, and he told her she still had some toxic metals remaining in her mouth.

According to Dr. Clark, the breakdown of metals in the mouth provides a slow and steady trickle of metals that poison the liver, bone marrow, thyroid, thymus, spleen, and parathyroids; these metals then slowly rob the body of good health. She explained that these organs have regulatory functions, which are needed by the body in order to regulate the levels of many different substances the body requires for good health. When these organs fail, there is death.

I read several testimonials of individuals who claimed to have miraculously recovered from cancer, as well as other degenerative diseases, within just a few weeks after having the dental metals removed. On the *Incurables,* a television program featuring individuals who have been healed of various diseases using alternative medicine, I saw accounts of people who had suffered with multiple sclerosis for years and were able to get out of wheelchairs and begin walking again only a few days after having the dental metals removed from their mouths.

The toxic seepage of metals is not the only problem created by dental metal work. Dental metal work is a breeding ground for a very dangerous bacterium known as Clostridium bacteria. The Clostridium bacteria hide and multiply in the crevices of metal dental work. The overuse of antibiotics has resulted in the Clostridium bacteria becoming a widespread problem. This illness is commonly known as C Diff; the C stands for Clostridium. A deficiency in the mineral iodine plays a major part in C Diff.

According to those who practice alternative medicine, conventional medicine has for years ignored the ability of iodine to destroy a bacterial or fungal infection, and instead choosing to treat with antibiotics. Gradually our modern diets have created a deficiency of iodine in the body. The recommended daily allowance of iodine for an adult is around 150 micrograms per day. I read the claims of a physician, who practices alternative medicine, that iodine deficiency is directly related to type II diabetes. Drinking chlorinated water, eating breads containing potassium bromide, as well as consuming too much sodium chloride, will inhibit the body from absorbing iodine and this eventually creates a deficiency in the body. The use of potassium bromide in manufacturing bread products is outlawed in other nations, but the FDA asks manufacturers to stop using potassium bromide on a volunteer basis here in the United States. It wasn't surprising to discover that other nations don't want our baked products either. Read the labeled ingredients and check for the presence of potassium chloride to protect your health.

I learned from Dr. Clark's writings that the Clostridium bacteria are responsible for causing tumors in the colon, which includes the mouth, the doorway to the colon. This is the most common way disease enters the body, through the mouth—first the colon where it becomes established and then metastasizing or spreading elsewhere. Small tumors may go undetected in the colon for years. I learned a cancerous tumor does not have to be large in order to metastasize or spread and find another place to establish itself. The cells just break away and travel; sometimes as the result of a blow or injury to the body or even a needle biopsy which breaks into an encapsulated tumor and allows cancerous cells to be released into the bloodstream.

Clostridium bacteria are commonly found in dairy products, and for this reason, dairy products should be sterilized by heat or treated with a couple of drops of 35% food grade hydrogen peroxide when a person is ill with cancer.

I watched another interview of a woman on the *Incurables* program, a woman who had battled Hodgkin's lymphoma for years. She was initially treated with conventional medicine and because she did not get any positive results, she resorted to alternative medicine, which included a complete change in her diet. Although she improved, she did not fully recover until she had her dental metals removed. A few days after having the dental metals removed, she was totally symptom-free and has continued to enjoy good health for many years.

Utilizing glass or enamel cookware rather than stainless steel, aluminum and nonstick cookware will aid in reducing exposure to toxic metals. Check second-hand stores for glass items. Since glass cookware is difficult to clean, it often ends up being donated to thrift shops. I read a study linking the development of the painful disease of osteoarthritis and the use of nonstick cookware.

Dr. Clark claimed the dangers of metals in the body are genuinely real. She said there are varieties of bacteria and yeast that attack our bodies only if nickel is present in the body. When the metal nickel is present, bacteria and yeast are then able to produce a toxic enzyme which enables these bacteria and yeast to thrive.

When heavy metals enter the body through the lungs, skin and digestive tract, they are swept along in the bloodstream as minute particles, lodging in the tissue of organs and settling or sinking into the lowest spot on the body, the lowest spot in the body, of course, being our feet. This is the reason why so many people suffer with toenail fungus. Dr. Clark claimed the most likely exposure to these offending metals is dental metal.

According to Dr. Clark, this tendency of the heavy metals to settle to the bottom also frequently occurs in the fingers, resulting in fungal infections in the fingernails.

Choose wooden, plastic, or rubber spoons and spatulas to cook with rather than metal, and if a person is extremely ill or experiencing a lot of pain, she said the use of plastic eating utensils can be an excellent choice. Completely avoid Styrofoam, as it is a known carcinogen which contains BPA, a hormone disruptor.

Dr. Clark warned against drinking or cooking with water taken from the hot water tap. The heating element from an electric hot water heater causes a release of heavy metals into the water. This happens with a gas hot water heater, as well. Heated water leaches metal from the pipes. Make sure you begin cooking with cold water from the tap and heat water on the stovetop in a glass vessel. Avoid using a microwave!

From Dr. Clark's book, I learned gold in or on the body could also cause a woman to suffer problems with her ovaries. I had a young friend who had her navel pierced, and she purchased a gold ring to wear in the pierce. I have to say, she rocked it, but not long after she started wearing the gold ring, she began to suffer with pain in one of her ovaries. She experienced some light vaginal bleeding and visited a gynecologist with her complaint. The gynecologist noted that her ovary was indeed inflamed and said they would have to keep an eye on it.

Not long after this, she came to see me for a few days and mentioned her visit with the doctor. When she lifted her blouse to show me the swelling over her ovary, I saw the gold ring. I shared with her gold is actually toxic to the body and can cause many women to experience ovarian problems. She removed the gold ring in her belly button immediately, with plans to purchase a plastic version. She awoke the following morning with no symptoms of pain or swelling in her ovary. Several months passed, and she informed me she had experienced no further problems with her ovary.

If a woman suffers with ovarian problems and she wears gold or other metal jewelry, she owes it to herself to set these things aside for a few days just to see whether her symptoms subside.

Switch to plastic eyewear, rather than metal frames, as this can be another source of metal seeping into the body. Every change that is made, large or small, can add up to restoring your health!

I learned the heavy metals and harmful chemicals we soak up from our environments serve to increase the level of acid in our bloodstream. As maintaining a pH of 7.36 to 7.44 is critical in getting the upper hand over cancer, we must become aware of the source of these acid-causing agents in order to take steps to avoid them. Our modern industrial world has the ability to saturate us with toxins, and it is for this reason we must learn what measures to take to routinely cleanse our bodies. If we neglect to do this, we will eventually pay the price for harboring substances which are detrimental to our health. I learned that drinking a few drops of 35% food grade hydrogen peroxide 3 times a day would safely increase the alkalinity in my bloodstream, increase the level of oxygen in my blood and increase my energy for just pennies a day.

In addition to the heavy metals and harmful chemicals encountered in our environments, as well as the presence of heavy metals in the herbicides and pesticides in our foods, and the mercury amalgam fillings we may have in our teeth, heavy metals are also commonly found in prescription drugs, as well as over-the-counter medications.

Again, the far infrared sauna and ion cleanse foot detox will aid in pulling these heavy metals from the body. I have seen hundreds of metal shards removed in one single ion cleanse foot detox administered to a person who had suffered with a street drug addiction for over a year. These metals are stored throughout the body, in the cells. If these metals are not cleansed from the body but are instead allowed to remain, microscopic amounts of these metals will eventually be given the opportunity to lodge in the brain, being carried there in the bloodstream. The very presence of these metals will adversely impact the memory, causing mental fogginess. Remember the presence of heavy metals anywhere in the body lends itself to fungal infection. There is no difference as to whether the metals are in the brain or the toes or places in between; fungus is the result.

Is this what dementia and Alzheimer's actually are—metals in the brain that result in fungus? I read that individuals who used a large number of drugs in their lifetime were more likely to develop dementia and Alzheimer's disease. If I had used a lot of drugs in my lifetime, this would prompt me to begin a program of daily detoxification.

With the understanding that heavy metals lead to fungus and fungus to cancer, it then becomes vitally important to relieve the body of heavy metals. Another effective way I read about that helps cleanse the body of heavy metals, which is also a very inexpensive solution, is taking food grade diatomaceous earth. This product can be located in the pet section of an independently owned health food store, as well as online. I read a few blogs posted by people who took a teaspoon in a glass of water or juice first thing in the morning. I learned it is important to avoid breathing diatomaceous earth, as it has the potential of damaging the lungs. Food grade diatomaceous earth dissolves in liquid easily. When I take diatomaceous earth, I just put it in a jar with a lid and shake it before drinking. Food grade diatomaceous earth will give you a big boost in energy and will keep you awake at night if you take it too late in the afternoon. It is important to take an adequate amount of wild source vitamin C when taking food grade diatomaceous earth. The vitamin C will help prevent constipation when using food grade diatomaceous earth.

One of the conditions a person can suffer with when they have an excess of heavy metals in the body or have been administered a lot of antibiotics is candida albicans. The illness of candida albicans is a breeding ground for the disease of cancer. It is perfectly normal for the body to have candida in the gut. However, antibiotics can trigger candida albicans to begin rapidly growing out of control. You can tell if you have a problem with candida albicans overgrowth by sticking your tongue out while looking into a mirror. If the back of your tongue is white, you most likely have a candida albicans overgrowth. There are many other symptoms which indicate a candida albicans overgrowth, among them being problems with bloating, flatulence, diarrhea, chronic constipation, and the appearance of small bumps on the sides of the arms. Also associated with this condition is a craving for sugar, refined carbohydrates and alcohol. See Chapter 22 for what I found as a solution when I developed an overgrowth of candida albicans.

If one has an occupation which exposes them to chemicals, their body can easily become burdened with heavy metals, making detoxification part of the daily routine an absolute necessity.

After recovering from breast cancer, I began searching for a local source of organic produce and spoke with a farmer located a few miles from our city. I was trying to locate organic strawberries at the time, and related my concern about chemicals being sprayed on food. He told me he had no organic strawberries. He said he had sprayed all of his fields surrounding his home with a fungicide. He then added he was currently in a battle with prostate cancer himself—not surprising at all—and being treated with estrogen therapy! He was living right in the middle of the reason he had cancer. The farmer was never going to get well while living in that environment.

There are many occupations, which expose us to toxins, and I learned those who are exposed to toxins on the job have to make detoxification a lifestyle habit if they want to remain healthy.

Another occupation, which typically exposes a person to heavy metals, is that of a hairdresser. Anyone with this occupation needs to take extra care in detoxifying the body on a regular basis. In addition to toxins increasing the likelihood of disease in the body, their presence will also produce estrogen dominance and result in the accumulation of stubborn body fat located primarily in the midsection. It is very typical for women who dye their hair to eventually store body fat in the midsection. Detoxification is the key to remaining healthy when you are a regular user of hair dye. Go to www.ibeatcancers.com to see a selection of available organic hair dye.

CHAPTER 16

Avoiding Dangerous Hormone Disruptors

My people are destroyed for a lack of knowledge.—Hosea 4:6

When I first learned of the threat hormone disruptors posed to my future health, I felt pretty overwhelmed and wondered whether I could even combat what was a real threat to my life. However, I learned I could still enjoy a normal life and that there were simple measures I could take which would aid in protecting my health. I have put together a list of the most common toxins which disrupt the hormones and have also included the steps I take to avoid them. These toxins can result in escalating the production of certain hormones in the body; reduce the production of others; mimic some hormones; cause one hormone to turn into another; hinder hormone signaling; cause cells to die prematurely; compete with essential nutrients; bind to essential hormones; and accumulate in organs which produce hormones. All of this means that the likelihood of developing or redeveloping hormonal cancer is increased when we are exposed to these hormone disruptors.

Below is a list which provides information on where these toxins are found and the steps I took to reduce exposure.

Dioxins: Dioxins form during numerous industrial processes when chlorine or bromine is burned in the presence of carbon and oxygen. Dioxins disrupt the delicate hormone signaling which occurs in the body of both males and females. Research has shown that exposure to low levels of dioxin in the womb and early in life can both permanently affect sperm quality and lower the sperm count in men during their prime reproductive years. Dioxins build up in the body and in the food chain. They are powerful carcinogens and can also affect the immune and reproductive systems.

How I reduced my exposure: As a result of the ongoing industrial discharge of dioxin, our food supply is widely contaminated with dioxins here in the U.S. Products including meat, fish, milk, eggs and butter are often affected; so going organic will make a difference. Dioxins are also present in commercial laundry detergent and enter the bloodstream through our constant skin contact with clothing, towels and sheets. See Chapter 27 on instructions for homemade laundry soap or see my website www.ibeatcancers.com for healthy laundry alternatives.

Atrazine: Researchers have learned that exposure to even low levels of the herbicide atrazine turned male frogs into females that produced viable eggs. Atrazine is regularly used on corn crops in the United States, and as a consequence, it is a commonplace contaminant in drinking water. This contaminant has been linked to breast tumors, delayed puberty and prostate inflammation in animals and some research has linked it to prostate cancer in men.

How I reduced my exposure: I always try to choose organic produce whenever possible. Avocadoes and bananas and the like are an exception because of their thick peel. Purchasing a drinking water filter certified to remove atrazine is a step in the right direction. To find a suitable filter check out www.ibeatcancers.com.

Phthalates: It is a little known fact that a specific signal programs cells in the body to die. It is completely normal for 50 billion cells in the body to die each day. Research has shown that chemicals called phthalates trigger what are known as *death-inducing signaling* in testicular cells, causing premature death of the cell. Researchers have linked phthalates to a low sperm count, less mobile sperm, hormonal changes, birth defects in the male reproductive system, obesity, diabetes, and thyroid irregularities.

How I reduced my exposure: I store food in glass containers, rather than plastics, and purchase plastic wrap which is BPA-free from the supermarket. Some personal care products contain phthalates, so I am a label reader and avoid products that list added *fragrance*; this is a commonly used term which most often means hidden phthalates. Find phthalate-free personal care products at www.ibeatcancers.com.

Lead: It is a well-known fact that lead is toxic. Lead harms almost every organ system in the body and has been linked to numerous health issues, including permanent brain damage, lowered IQ, hearing loss, miscarriage, premature birth, increased blood pressure, kidney damage and nervous system problems. However, few people realize that one other way in which lead may affect the body is by disrupting hormones. In animals, lead has been found to lower sex hormone levels. Research shows that lead disrupts hormone signaling.

How I reduced my exposure: Old paint is a major source of lead exposure and should be removed professionally. I purchased a good water filter to reduce exposure to lead in my drinking water. Find one at www.ibeatcancers.com. Using a cast iron cooking vessel will aid in combatting lead exposure. Research has found that a healthy diet reduces lead absorption.

Polybrominated diphenyl ethers: This contaminant was first identified by researchers in women's breast milk in 1972 and has been detected in increasing levels in breast milk ever since. This contaminant, commonly known as PBDEs, has been found in the tissue of people and wildlife around the globe – even polar bears. PBDEs imitate thyroid hormones in the body and disrupt their activity. Although the use of some PBDEs has been discontinued, their presence has not been reduced because they do not break down in the environment.

How I reduced my exposure: I learned to always use a vacuum cleaner with a HEPA filter, as this will cut down on toxic-laden house dust. Avoid reupholstering old foam furniture. As the padding underneath your old carpet may contain PBDE's, have it removed by a professional and replaced with a suitable product. I switched to tile and now rely on area rugs.

Perchlorate: Perchlorate is a component in rocket fuel, so it is not surprising to learn that this is a contaminant found in produce and milk; even organic products are contaminated with perchlorates, as jet fuel is not discriminating when it is dispersed into the atmosphere. When perchlorate gets into the body it competes with the nutrient iodine. This is known as displacement. The thyroid gland needs iodine to make thyroid hormones.

This means that ingesting too much of it can alter the thyroid hormone balance. These hormones regulate metabolism in adults and are crucial for proper brain and organ development in infants and young children.

How I reduced my exposure: Perchlorate in drinking water can be filtered by reverse osmosis filter. Check the wide selection of water filters and distillers available on my website by going to www.ibeatcancers.com. I learned it's impossible to avoid perchlorate in my food, but its potential effects on the body can be reduced by making sure I'm getting enough iodine in my diet. I use an iodine supplement, but not every day. Iodine is also found in kelp tablets, kelp, seafood and iodized salt. I learned that as a woman, inadequate levels of iodine in the body leads to hair loss and obesity.

BPA: BPA is a chemical used in plastics and actually imitates the sex hormone estrogen in the body. Unfortunately, because the body recognizes BPA as estrogen, it stores it. BPA has been linked to everything from breast and others cancers to reproductive problems, obesity, early puberty and heart disease, and according to government released testing, 93 percent of Americans are storing BPA in their bodies!

How I reduced my exposure: I eat fresh rather than canned food. Many food cans are lined with BPA. Look for labeling that indicates BPA-free – or a similar chemical – in their packaging in order to avoid this toxin. Say no to receipts, since thermal paper is often coated with BPA. I ask that the receipt be put into a bag and remove it later while wearing a latex glove. Avoid plastics marked with a "PC," for polycarbonate, or recycling label #7. Not all of these plastics contain BPA, but many do – and it is important to keep synthetic hormones out of the body. Some little known places where BPA can be found: Pizza boxes, recycled paper, toilet paper (Charmin makes a BPA-free product), receipts, wine fermented in BPA-resin lined vats, beer similarly processed, Rubbermaid baking tins used by Subway, soda cans, organic canned tomatoes, common plastic cups, blue-tinted hard plastic drinking water bottles, leak-free paper plates, and I'm sorry to say the list goes on.

Arsenic: In large enough amounts, arsenic will kill. In smaller amounts, the ingestion of arsenic can result in skin, bladder and lung cancer. Arsenic can interfere with normal hormone functioning in the glucocorticoid system that regulates how our bodies process sugars and carbohydrates. This means overexposure to arsenic is linked to weight gain or loss, suppression of the immune system, insulin resistance, osteoporosis, growth retardation and high blood pressure.

How I reduced my exposure: I learned wild source vitamin C helps to protect the body from arsenic. I also learned I could reduce my exposure by using a water filter that lowers arsenic levels. For help finding wild source vitamin C, go to www.ibeatcancers.com.

Mercury: Sushi may be hazardous to your health. Mercury is a naturally occurring but toxic metal. The foremost way mercury enters the air and the oceans is through burning coal. Eventually, mercury can appear on the dining table in the form of mercury-contaminated seafood. Those who are at the highest risk of the toxic effects of mercury are pregnant women, since the metal is known to concentrate in the fetal brain and interferes with brain development. Mercury is also known to interfere with fertility, as it binds directly to one particular hormone which regulates a woman's menstrual cycle and ovulation. Mercury has been shown to damage cells in the pancreas that produce insulin, which is critical for the body's ability to metabolize sugar, which means it may very well promote the disease of diabetes.

How I reduced my exposure: I love wild salmon and learned that Curcumin, also known as the spice turmeric, and selenium protect the body from the toxic effects of mercury. Wow, these two nutrients are anti-cancer! I used to always reach for the Pacific wild salmon, but the radiation which has reached Alaska's shores from Japan's Fukushima nuclear plant accident may very well make this a poor choice. I don't know this for a fact, but it makes sense to me. I now select farm-raised salmon from Scotland.

Perfluorinated chemicals (PFCs): The perfluorinated chemicals used to make non-stick cookware can stick to you. Perfluorinated chemicals are so widespread that it is estimated 99 percent of the American population has these chemicals in their bodies. One compound called PFOA has been shown to completely resist biodegradation. In other words, PFOA doesn't break down in the environment – ever. This means that even though the chemical was banned after decades of use, it will continue to be present for generations to come. PFOA exposure has been linked to decreased sperm quality, low birth weight, kidney disease, thyroid disease and high cholesterol, among other health issues. Scientists are still figuring out how

PFOA affects the human body. Animal studies have shown that it affects thyroid and sex hormone levels.

How I reduced my exposure: I stopped using non-stick pans; this was a very difficult choice for me. After all, all the great cooks on television use non-stick pans. I now stick to cast iron and stainless steel, no pun intended. I also learned it was important to avoid stain and water-resistant coatings on clothing, furniture and carpets.

Organophosphate pesticides: These neurotoxic compounds were produced by the Nazis in huge quantities for chemical warfare during World War II. Fortunately they were never used. However, after the war ended, German-owned pharmaceutical companies used the same chemistry to develop a long line of pesticides that target the nervous systems of insects. Despite the many studies linking exposure to organophosphate, which include effects on brain development, behavior and fertility, they are still commonly used today. Organophosphates can affect the human body by interfering with the way testosterone communicates with cells, lowering testosterone and altering thyroid hormone levels.

How I reduced my exposure: I buy organic whenever possible.

Glycol Ethers: Researchers have found that when male rats are exposed to glycol ethers, their testicles shrink. Glycol ethers are common solvents in paints, cleaning products, brake fluid and cosmetics. The European Union says that some of these chemicals "may damage fertility or the unborn child." Studies of painters have linked exposure to certain glycol ethers to blood abnormalities and lower sperm counts. And children who were exposed to glycol ethers from paint in their bedrooms had substantially more asthma and allergies.

How I reduced my exposure: Check Chapter 27 for healthy cleaning alternatives and go to www.ibeatcancers.com to find non-toxic cosmetics.

CHAPTER 17

Fossil Fuel Pollutants

Heaven and earth shall pass away, but my words
shall not pass away.—Matthew 24:35

I read an article in my local newspaper with regard to a government study. The article stated something we most likely all realized before the government poured only-God-knows-how-much of the taxpayers' hard earned cash into the study: Breathing gasoline and diesel fumes while stuck in traffic is toxic to the body. The conclusion of the study was fossil fuel fumes were estrogenic and caused cancer. Along with these estrogens, breathing these fumes also pulls heavy metals into the body. We instinctively realize breathing these fumes cannot possibly be beneficial. I'm sure I'm not the only one who has tried to hold her breath as a city bus lumbered past, belching out billowing clouds of pollutants.

Other than moving out to the fresh air of the country to escape the fumes or relocating to a city where electric mass transportation is the norm, we all experience this unavoidable evil. Little can be done to remedy this; however, according to Dr. Clark, there is something we can do about cleaning up our immediate environments; and this can make a dramatic difference in our ability to recover our health.

We can begin by removing all gasoline and noxious chemical products from our home and garage. If the garage is attached to the house, avoid parking the car in the garage. According to Dr. Clark, fumes leak from our cars and seep into the home, as well as polluting the air in the garage which is often a daily passageway. (After I got well, I put my car back into the garage.) Remove the lawnmower and all other gasoline-powered equipment—weed whacker, blower, edger, hedge trimmer, and chain saw. Remove gasoline cans and all petroleum products from the environment.

The air in the garage should be fresh and not tax or burden the immune system. These very necessary changes allow the immune system relief from battling pollutants while one sits in their home! Sleeping in a room that is next to a garage full of carcinogens increases your chances of developing cancer, and this also applies to sleeping in a room that is above a garage that is harboring these contaminants.

These changes may require investing in an exterior storage shed or discarding certain items altogether, but your health is at stake.

If you have any propane gas lines leading into the home for kitchen appliances or are heating water or your home with a propane gas heater, have a professional check these lines annually. If you indeed have a propane gas leak in the home, this can very well be the origin of a cancerous tumor.

SECTION 3

Steps I Took to Get Well

CHAPTER 18

Preparing for the Cancer Remedy

How God anointed Jesus of Nazareth, who went
about doing good and healing all...- Acts 10:38

As I have stated before, I am not a physician, and I possess no medical training. Therefore, I am unqualified to prescribe medical remedies or any sort of treatment for cancer or any other disease. The dosages I have listed below and in other chapters are what worked for me, but glory, hallelujah, they worked very quickly and wonderfully well. I took what was recommended by Dr. Clark for an adult.

Unlike the cancer remedies prescribed by conventional medicine, nothing I took made me feel ill. Aside from the cold I developed as the result of detoxification illness when I took the Juice of Wild Oreganol to combat breast cancer, everything I took made me feel better!

In preparing my body to take the cancer remedy, I began by taking 5 drops of Lugol's iodine in 6 ounces of water each morning. I sipped it through a straw so it did not discolor my teeth. I only did this for a week and then took it 3 times a week. I learned I needed to avoid eating dairy products 2 hours before and after taking iodine, as well as completely avoiding raw cruciferous vegetables, as these two food groups would negate the effectiveness of iodine. I learned I could skip this step if I was allergic to iodine. I also learned that if I was unsure of whether I had an iodine allergy, that I could apply a small test patch of iodine on the inside of my upper arm. If I had not developed a rash by the next day, I could safely take iodine.

Following my morning dose of iodine, I began taking what I call the detox trio, three capsules of wild source rose hip vitamin C, two capsules of hydrangea root, and three capsules of selenium, as recommended by Dr. Clark in her book, *The Cure & Prevention of all Cancers*. These products are available on my website, www.ibeatcancers.com.

I learned taking these three supplements is vitally important, as they boost the immune system and help prevent the development of pneumonia. Pneumonia can develop because the breakdown of the tumor introduces many harmful toxins into the bloodstream. If the supplements in the detox trio are not present in the body, these harmful toxins go to the lungs, which is the body's attempt at detoxifying through the lungs.

Wild source vitamin C stimulates the production of white blood cells in the immune system, and the increase of the white blood cell count allows the body to prevail over the disease of cancer. Selenium helps the white blood cells get rid of yeast in the body. Yeast feeds cancer.

Ideally, I learned it is best to take the detox trio for a few days before commencing with either the eighteen day herbal germ cleanse or the Juice of Wild Oreganol. I realized I had an emergency on my hands and neglected to take the detox trio for the first few days. Failing to begin with the detox trio is most likely the reason I developed a deep chest cold and possibly pneumonia, as the toxins went to my lungs instead of being flushed through my kidneys.

The immune system is comprised of a beautifully complex system of cells, and whether or not someone survives cancer depends on the strength of the immune system.

This means taking the rose hip vitamin C, hydrangea root, and selenium is crucial, as these three supplements enable the white blood cells to release toxins into the kidneys, where they are passed on to the bladder and leave the body through urination.

I purchased the following supplements from the Dr. Clark Store.

MY MORNING DOSE OF THE DETOX TRIO

3 capsules of rose hip vitamin C; I took the one which had 550 mg. per capsule
2 capsules of hydrangea root
3 capsules of selenium.

Without the detox trio the white blood cells of the immune system cannot release toxins into the kidneys. According to Dr. Clark, the white blood cells need to be unburdened of toxins so they are free to get back to work again. Simply put, taking the detox trio was essential to my healing process. See Chapter 10 for a simple method to help rebuild the immune system.

Once the white blood cells are relieved of the toxins they have been carting around, they are free to gobble up the substantial amount of toxins produced when taking an herbal germ cleanse. According to Dr. Clark, the dying cancerous tumor will send a whole slew of contaminants into the colon, toxins which she warns can cause a person to develop pneumonia.

I learned the detox trio should be taken once a day, in the morning, followed by additional doses of rose hip vitamin C throughout the day, one or two capsules at a time, as many as three to four times daily, whatever can be tolerated by my bowels. I learned I must drink plenty of water when I take vitamin C. Too much vitamin C will produce diarrhea so I learned to work up to higher dosages gradually and not to neglect eating fiber on a daily basis. I ate a small amount of fiber mixed in with each meal, such as a teaspoon of ground flax seed, chia seeds or Psyllium husk. These fibers required me to drink a great deal of water throughout the day, which is excellent because water aids in flushing the body of toxins. Fiber reduces the risk of diarrhea, as it soaks up the liquid in the colon, allowing for stool formation.

Likewise, if I experienced constipation, I learned vitamin C is an excellent remedy to move the bowels, with the added benefit of strengthening the cells.

Very important: I swallowed the capsules one at a time. If I needed to, I could eat a little something to prevent the capsules from sticking in my throat. I learned that if I needed to I could open the capsules and mix the contents with food to make taking them easier. It was not required that I take the detox trio on an empty stomach.

CHAPTER 19

An Eighteen-Day Herbal Germ Cleanse

I sought the Lord, and He heard me, and delivered
me from all of my fears —Psalm 34:4

The very first day I began this germ cleanse, I felt a noticeable improvement in my health. I found these products to be powerful and effective. These products eliminate dangerous microbes in the body that Dr. Clark associated with the disease of cancer. Dr. Clark claimed that these products could reverse the health of someone who was "on their deathbed."

The products she recommended include black walnut tincture or capsules, wormwood capsules and clove capsules. These are products produced by the Dr. Clark Store and are available at www.ibeatcancers.com.

When I purchased these herbs, I also purchased the supplement ornithine. This chapter also includes Dr. Clark's suggested instructions on the need and use of ornithine. Chapter 36 provides a list of products I used to get well.

USER GUIDE

DAY	Black Walnut Hull Extra Strength: Take either the liquid tincture or the capsules	Wormwood Capsules	Clove Capsules
1	1 drop or 1 pinch of powder	1 cap	1·1·1
2	2 drops or 2 pinches of powder	1 cap	2·2·2
3	3 drops or 3 pinches of powder	2 caps	3·3·3
4	4 drops or 4 pinches of powder	2 caps	3·3·3
5	5 drops or 1 capsule	3 caps	3·3·3
6	2 tsp. or 5 capsules	3 caps	3·3·3
7	None	4 caps	3·3·3
8	None	4 caps	3·3·3
9	None	5 caps	3·3·3
10	None	5 caps	3·3·3
11	None	6 caps	7 caps all at once
12	None	6 caps	None
13	2 tsp. / 5 capsules	7 caps	None
14	None	7 caps	None
15	None	7 caps	None
16	None	7 caps	None
17	None	7 caps	None
18	None	7 caps	7 caps all at once

Dr. Clark recommends a person diagnosed with terminal cancer drink a lot of black walnut tincture (even an entire bottle in a single day when the diagnosis is terminal) frequently sipping it throughout the day, making sure to take the combination of black walnut, wormwood, and clove capsules also. I learned taking things very, very slowly helps avoid the feeling of being nauseated. I also learned about Dr. Clark's recommendation of following up the herbal germ cleanse with a gallbladder/liver flush. Instructions for the flush are included in the chapter entitled "The Cleanup Program." Dr. Clark placed a great deal of emphasis on completing this flush within two days of finishing the herbal germ cleanse. I learned that if I had been very ill, it would be best to wait until I was stronger.

However, I learned it would be a good idea to do daily enemas with warm water and 2 ounces of Miracle II Neutralizer until I felt stronger.

I learned drinking small amounts of the Miracle II products during this cleanse could be helpful, as well as using them while bathing. Miracle

II products come with a User Guide. To begin with, the company recommends taking 3 drops of Miracle II soap and 7 drops of Miracle II Neutralizer in a glass of water on a daily basis. The taste is not unpleasant. The Miracle II products aid in washing the body on the inside!

If I decide to do an herbal germ cleanse now, I now do a very quick cleanse of 5 capsules of black walnut, 7 capsules of wormwood and 7 capsules of cloves, all at once on an empty stomach,15 minutes before eating, taking this amount for a week.

When a person is terminally ill, though, the process has to be much slower because the toxic die-off will produce illness. I learned from Dr. Clark's book that a gradual approach will produce much better results.

In addition to the above, I took the following doses of ornithine at night to combat insomnia. In the follow-up herbal germ cleanses I took I found I only needed to take ornithine the first night.

ORNITHINE TO RELIEVE INSOMNIA

First night	2 capsules
Second night	4 capsules
Third night	6 capsules

I continued taking six ornithine capsules each night if I experienced any sleeplessness, and I did experience insomnia initially, so I found it is extremely important to have ornithine on hand. I learned the die-off of toxins results in the production of ammonia in the body. When this ammonia circulates into the brain, insomnia is the result.

I found the supplement arginine will help to increase the energy level during the day while taking the herbal cleanse. I did not experience a loss of energy and did not take arginine, but I learned if I had experienced energy loss, I could take five hundred milligrams of arginine once in the morning and once at lunchtime. Since coffee should be avoided, arginine will help combat the sluggish feeling a former coffee drinker might experience in the morning.

I took the herbal germ cleanse remedy every day for 18 days and also used the apricot kernels, the product I discuss in the chapter entitled "The Mighty Apricot Seed." Taking apricot seeds during the herbal germ cleanse will increase the die-off of toxins. If a person has been sick with cancer for a long time, it is not recommended by Dr. Clark that they take more than one cancer remedy at a time.

I learned the herbal germ cleanse could be safely taken every three to six months, and even more frequently if I felt it necessary. During the 18-day herbal cleanse, I learned the importance of enemas or having a few colonic hydrotherapy procedures. I talk about this extensively in my chapter on "Bowel Health."

I learned from a doctor who practices alternative medicine that having a colonic hydrotherapy procedure performed by a colonic specialist would be a wise approach to take if suffering with constipation, as this would be a quick and efficient way to remove toxins from the colon and thus prevent detox illness.

Detox illness is the result of cancer cell die-off. Taking these powerful herbs will produce an overabundance of bacteria that must be removed from the colon as quickly as possible in order to prevent the bacteria from moving into the lungs and putting a person at risk for pneumonia. The colonic hydrotherapy also assists the lymphatic system in draining more efficiently, thus helping to speed the removal of dangerous toxins. I learned it would be best to wait a few days after first beginning the herbal cleanse to have a colonic, as the colonic procedure will decrease the effectiveness of the herbal germ cleanse. When a person suffers with colon cancer, I learned a colonic can actually be extremely helpful. The cost of a colonic procedure should be around $65.

I learned that taking Clear Lungs Extra Strength by Ridgecrest Herbals, a powerful and effective blend of Chinese herbal medicine, during the herbal germ cleanse will help prevent the bacteria produced in the germ die-off from settling into the lungs, thus preventing the development of pneumonia.

I was unaware of the danger the die-off posed to my health, and I did develop a deep chest cold, possibly even pneumonia. I was able to recover by taking Clear Lungs Extra Strength, two capsules several times a day. I tried other products, but Clear Lungs was the only thing that worked for me.

It is recommended to take two capsules of Clear Lungs made by Ridgecrest twice daily, but I learned they could be taken more frequently if a cold begins to develop as a result of the body quickly detoxifying. I only had to take them for a few days. If I was to go through this process again, I would purchase a nasal spray, such as one made with grapefruit seed extract to use as a preventative; just using it for the first week. I also learned of a nasal spray comprised of spices, a product of the North American Herb & Spice Company, that I could use for just a week during the herbal germ cleanse, as well. This discourages harmful bacteria in the airways. I also learned a colloidal silver product sprayed in the throat would aid in minimizing a cold or preventing a cold from getting established.

Dr. Clark wrote that this powerful herbal germ cleanse was effective in treating the HIV/AIDS virus. She did not claim this would cure the virus, but that it would most certainly improve the well-being of the patient. I learned that there were products which build the immune system, such as beta mannan produced by Alotek and beta glucan produced by NSC Immunition, which would also improve the condition of anyone who was suffering with an illness because these two products help to rebuild the immune system. Dr. Clark recommended the eighteen-day cleanse be used by persons suffering with Lyme's disease, as well as a multitude of other degenerative diseases.

I learned that detoxification using the far infrared sauna was extremely useful in remaining free from disease. When I was diligent about using the sauna, I found it was unnecessary to repeatedly use the herbal germ cleanse.

See Chapter 22 and learn about the amazing results I experienced from the use of 35% food grade hydrogen peroxide.

A person who is extremely ill will most likely be unable to tolerate a sauna initially. In this case, an alternative approach of detoxification is an ion cleanse foot detox, used during the herbal germ cleanse. Detoxification equipment and the herbal germ cleanse are available on my website, www. ibeatcancers.com. There is a great selection of equipment available: ion cleanse foot detox equipment, energy frequency machines, far infrared saunas, ozonating equipment, distillers, alkaline water equipment, showerheads that filter chlorine, and many other products that aid in remaining healthy.

Dr. Clark said it was perfectly safe to use the detoxification products, i.e., the Juice of Wild Oreganol, the herbal germ cleanse, and apricot kernels on the very same day or throughout the 18 days of cleansing. However, she emphasized it was important to remember the body would detox very quickly as a result. I learned that if I was really sick, the best approach would be to take it very slowly and patiently. Otherwise, I could possibly suffer horribly with nausea. So I learned to be cautious and not be overly enthusiastic, but to begin with the small doses, taking it slow and steady.

CHAPTER 20

The Cleanup Program

For thou hast girded me with strength unto the
battle: thou hast subdued under me those that
rose up against me.—Psalm 18:39 KJV

The next step is what Dr. Clark referred to as the cleanup or mop-up program, and this step involves cleansing the kidneys with her prescribed kidney cleansing herbal formula, followed by a gallbladder/liver flush. These steps were called very necessary by Dr. Clark. The kidney cleansing herbal formula prescribed by Dr. Clark should be taken before undertaking a liver flush.

The gallbladder/liver flush is intended to flush out of the body any harmful organisms that may remain after completion of the anti-cancer herbal cleanse. I learned this flush should be followed by a colonic hydrotherapy for best results. I also learned that I should not attempt this flush if I had been very ill. The gallbladder/liver flush is recommended by Dr. Clark and by several other physicians whose books I read. However, I also read that people should take caution using this flush. I learned of an easier flush that is not quite as harsh that I will share first. This quick liver flush would be more tolerable for someone who has been very ill.

QUICK LIVER FLUSH

This liver flush comes highly recommended as a remarkable drink with amazing rejuvenative properties. It reportedly increases energy, rapidly improves digestion, aids in cleansing the lymphatic system, normalizes saliva pH values and helps persons who are underweight to gain weight. It was claimed that with almost any chronic condition, this drink will have a beneficial effect. It was also reported that persons who are overweight will not gain weight on this drink.

To make the drink, take one whole lemon, seeds, flesh and rind and cut it up and place in a blender; a Nutribullet works great for this. Add 1 and ½ cups of distilled water or fruit juice and I tablespoon of extra virgin olive oil (cold pressed); then adding ¼ teaspoon of Himalayan pink salt. Blend this mixture at high speed for one minute. Pass the solution through a strainer and remove the pulp. Drink in 2 or 3 portions throughout the day. Take it before, during or after meals. It was recommended that you drink this solution as often as you like.

DR. CLARK'S LIVER FLUSH

The following items are necessary for this revitalizing gallbladder/ liver flush:

- 4 tablespoons of Epsom salts
- ½ cup of ozonated olive oil
- 2 large pink grapefruit
- 25 drops of black walnut tincture
- 1 orange or lemon sliced

Mix 4 tablespoons of Epsom salts and 3 cups of distilled water in a jar that has a lid. Refrigerate the jar of mixture until it is well chilled. You now have 4 servings of ¾ cup each.

Follow this schedule throughout the day. You may begin earlier or later, but make sure you adjust the times to follow the same time intervals.

Gallbladder/Liver Flush Schedule

7:00 a.m.: Drink ¾ cup of cold Epsom salts. Bite into a slice of citrus, such as an orange, lemon or grapefruit right after drinking.

9:00 a.m.: Drink ¾ cup of cold Epsom salts.

10:45 a.m.: Pour ½ cup of olive oil in a pint jar. Squeeze and strain a fresh grapefruit. This should make approximately ¾ cup of grapefruit juice. Mix the grapefruit juice with the ½ cup of olive oil and add 25 drops of black walnut tincture. Shake the mixture until it appears watery.

11:00 a.m.: Drink the solution within five minutes of preparation. Immediately lie down flat on your back, with your head propped up on a pillow. Keep perfectly still for at least 20 minutes. You might possibly experience the sensation of stones traveling along the bile ducts. It will be necessary to visit the bathroom and evacuate your bowels frequently. It would be best to keep a large absorbent towel between your legs just in case you don't quite make it to the toilet.

3:00 p.m.: Drink 7 to 8 ounces of distilled water.

6:00 p.m.: Drink ¾ cup of cold Epsom salts and go back to bed.

8:00 p.m.: Drink ¾ cup of cold Epsom salts. This is the final dose.

10:00 p.m.: Eat fruit or drink fresh fruit juice. It is recommended you drink 7.5 ounces of prune juice mixed with 2.5 ounces of distilled water.

10:30 p.m.: Eat cooked or raw fruit.

Expect to make many trips to the bathroom throughout the day and during the night. This flush will cause the undigested fats which burden the liver to be expelled from the body through the bowels, as well as expelling cancer-causing germs. By mid-morning the following day, the effects of the flush will be gone. You may feel tired and a little weak the second day, which is why this flush is best done over the weekend or during a couple of days when you have nothing else planned.

For optimum results, it is best to eat light meals of cooked and raw fruits for breakfast, steamed vegetables for lunch and fish and salad for dinner. Eating a heavy meal would defeat the long term purpose of the flush, in addition to very likely contributing to a lot of discomfort in the bowels.

This gallbladder/liver flush will leave you refreshed and energized within a couple of days. NOTE: It is important to remember the gallbladder/liver flush should not be repeated more frequently than every two weeks.

Dr. Clark also stressed the necessity of an ozonator as part of cleansing your system, as well as maintaining a healthy body. I found purchasing an ozonator to be very useful to my new lifestyle. I often ozonate the water I drink. The ozonator infuses oxygen into the water, and the oxygen purifies and energizes the body, as the body uses oxygen to create life and energy flow.

I found the ozonator to be a valuable and money-saving tool, as I can use the ozonator to clean non-organic produce, as it will remove chemicals, germs and bacteria, such as listeria and E. coli. I simply place the produce into a bucket full of water and place the aerator at the bottom of the bucket, then ozonate the contents for 7 minutes. After ozonating the submerged produce, I add one drop of Lugol's iodine per one quart of water in the bucket of water and allow the produce to sit submerged in the water for 1 minute before washing. The ozone has power to penetrate and destroy germs; the Lugol's iodine, on the other hand, has "attaching" ability. I learned each process has its own special value. I make sure to thoroughly rinse the produce before eating.

According to Dr. Clark, ozonating non-organic dairy products or meats for 15 minutes will destroy any estrogens, making it suitable for consumption; and the noxious effect of dyes that have been sprayed on meats will be destroyed if ozonated for 15 to 20 minutes. She said to place the food I wish to ozonate into a zip lock bag, place the aerator into the bag and zip it closed. When there is a buildup of pressure, the ozonated air will penetrate the food or beverage. I run the ozonator for the prescribed amount of time and allow the food to remain in the bag after turning off the ozonator. I allow the food to sit in the closed container for 10 more minutes before removing. Ozonating foods can alter the taste considerably, and Dr. Clark recommends using spices to improve the taste.

When I remove the detachable aerator and plastic tubing, the ozonator becomes a useful air purifier, as it quickly removes odors from the air. I found it is very effective in removing wet paint fumes and new carpet odors. Whenever I purchase new bedding which has a polyurethane odor -- polyurethane is a substance Dr. Clark linked to lung cancer, so, here again, an ozonator is a very useful item -- I create a tent over the article with a sheet and place the ozonator inside the tent. I simply turn it on for one hour, and repeat the process until the odor is gone. Polyurethane is very often an ingredient in items such as paint, foam mattresses, sealant and foam insulation. The fumes these products emit are dangerous and especially dangerous to people who are suffering with cancer.

The ozonator is useful in removing the noxious chemical fumes from dry cleaned clothing. I remove the plastic cover, hang it in a closet, put the ozonator inside the closet, turn it on, and close the closet door. I have used it to remove the new car odor from a vehicle, fumes which are linked to cancer. I was also successful in removing a lingering and very pungent fish odor from my husband's SUV, caused when he spilled an ice chest full of fish in his vehicle following a fishing trip. He was impressed!

Ozonating will also effectively clean surfaces in 20 minutes and quickly removes the odor of chlorine bleach.

Dr. Clark mentioned using an ozonator in the treatment of breast cancer. She recommended taping a clean plastic bag over the breast using clear packing tape. Tuck the ozonator aerator tip inside the bag and run the ozonator for 30 minutes. She said to leave the bag on for another 30 minutes before removing. Dr. Clark recommended that you leave the bag taped to the breast and repeat the process throughout the day. I did not do this but instead used the castor oil pack. The Juice of Wild of Oreganol, coupled with the right diet, was so effective for me that I did not really need to do anything else, and I later learned drinking 35% H202 was a wonderful way to supplement oxygen.

CHAPTER 21

Bowel Health

Your enemies shall come out against you one way and
flee before you seven ways.—Deuteronomy 28:7

I learned it was absolutely crucial to my recovery to have a bowel movement
at least once a day, preferably twice or, even better, three times. When
body waste is not eliminated on a daily basis, there is a rapid increase
in bacteria and fungus in the bowel, which burdens the organs and the
immune system, leaving the body's defenses weakened and more easily
challenged by disease.

Aside from constipation being a miserable experience which subjects
your bloodstream to toxins, constipation takes a toll on good health in
other ways. Constipation hinders the functions of the entire body. When
constipation is present, the lymphatic system becomes sluggish and does
not properly drain; the lymphatic system is then harboring toxins and
a feeling of lethargy is the result. While over-the-counter laxatives may
provide some relief, these products upset the delicate balance of good
bacteria present in the low gut, and serve to compromise the immune
system and should be taken in conjunction with the detox trio. Using these
products on a regular basis actually disarms the immune system, making
the body vulnerable to disease.

I learned a much better solution for constipation is to eat more
vegetables on a daily basis, vigilantly take the detox trio, use products
which contain fiber as well as probiotics, and drink an adequate amount
of water. Regular exercise is a must if I am to enjoy bowel regularity and

good health. I have read that as little as 15 minutes a day is a sufficient amount of exercise to provide a favorable impact on health.

Many people religiously have a colonoscopy exam each year as a preventative health care measure. Although the colonoscopy allows for the removal of pre-cancerous polyps, a quick search on the Internet will reveal numerous examples of colonoscopies gone awry as the result of a faulty sterilization process. I learned this procedure has exposed thousands of people to hepatitis C and HIV as well as other diseases, fungi, and bacteria. This is an invasive procedure which is undoubtedly highly profitable for the medical community.

I learned from reading Dr. Clark's writings that the first line of defense in preventing colon cancer is to keep the mouth clean. Because Clostridium bacteria are invasive bacteria that are harbored in the crevices of dental metal in the mouth, good dental hygiene will aid in preventing disease. Clostridium bacterium is the bacteria responsible for the development of tumors in the mouth, throat, colon, rectum, and lymphatic system, according to Dr. Clark. This insidious bacterium is present in dairy products, thus making the sterilization of dairy products for anyone with a challenged immune system of vital importance.

I learned from Dr. Clark that Clostridium bacteria are easily contracted from handling your pet. For this reason, it is very important to wash your hands thoroughly after having contact with a pet. It is also important to never allow pets to lick your face. Likewise, washing hands after using the bathroom is crucial. I learned the Juice of Wild Oreganol, which kills the Clostridium bacteria, will prevent these tumors from forming and quickly rid the body of tumors which may already be established.

It is suggested you take the Juice of Wild Oreganol three times a day, holding it in the mouth for as long as possible before swallowing. In our home, we keep it alongside the products we use for dental care, making sure each time we brush our teeth, we take a mouthful of the Juice of Wild Oreganol. Now, that is what constitutes a sensible preventative measure to insure colon health.

Dr. Clark suggested that taking Betaine hydrochloride, 1500 mg. twice a day, would also protect from the dangerous effects of Clostridium bacteria, stopping diarrhea in its tracks. As the result of my successful battle against cancer, I began reading with interest what Dr. Clark had written regarding the effects of bacteria in the body and the natural solutions which were available. It was during this particular time we had a month-long houseguest, who had brought along a couple of large dogs. One of the dogs developed diarrhea that went on for days; it was difficult, to say the least.

The dog's master surmised her pet had most likely eaten the feces left by a wild animal in our yard. Our houseguest asked me to suggest a good veterinarian in the area. My newly found knowledge led me to suspect the dog had contracted the Clostridium bacteria, and I suggested we first try a home remedy of Betaine hydrochloride. She gave the large dog a 500 mg. capsule. The dog vomited the first capsule, but then her owner decided to give it another try, and the dog kept down the second capsule. After a single dose, one capsule, the dog made a full recovery that very day.

From Dr. Clark's book, I learned to take one capsule of Betaine hydrochloride with a meal, as it greatly aids the function of the pancreas and improves digestion. As useful as Betaine hydrochloride is, it does not provide the exact same benefits as the Juice of Wild Oreganol. The Juice of Wild Oreganol has a very strong taste and may not be tolerated by some people. I give it to my husband in a vegetable juice mixture to help disguise the strong taste, making it more tolerable. I do know of people who give their dogs Oreganol Oil capsules every day disguised in a treat, and this would be a great preventative for a pet against the Clostridium bacteria.

The mouth is the entrance to the colon, and when the mouth is kept clean, colon health will naturally improve; having the proper balance of healthy bacteria in the low gut is of equal importance.

I learned to avoid using commercial mouthwash which can contain isopropyl alcohol, dyes, and other toxins. I now use a diluted solution of food grade hydrogen peroxide as a mouthwash. This solution removes stains and provides for a beautiful smile.

Dr. Clark suggested that toothpaste often negatively interacts with dental metal work. I learned to brush my teeth with aluminum-free baking soda and a drop of clove oil. The North American Herb & Spice Company sells clove oil as Clovenol. A drop of Clovenol on a hurting tooth will ease the pain very quickly.

I also learned that you could treat inflammation in the gums with myrrh, as it is extremely effective in drawing the infection out of the gums, and it is not dangerous if swallowed, rather it is healing to the gut. I was advised to hold the myrrh in my mouth as long as possible, swishing it around for at least a few minutes before spitting it out.

There is another approach that can be used to help detox the body through the mouth. This is the practice known as oil pulling and should be performed the very first thing in the morning. These are the instructions I was given: Take one tablespoon of a good quality coconut oil, and begin to swish it back and forth with the tongue while keeping the jaws relaxed. Do not hold the head back or attempt to gargle, as the oil will begin to seep down the throat. Do this very gently, back and forth, for twenty minutes, and then spit the oil out. This is most effective when done on an empty stomach first thing in the morning.

I learned the colon plays a vital part in the body's ability to heal, as its role is to absorb the nutrients from the food, rid the body of waste matter, and eliminate toxins which accumulate in the body. If the colon is not healthy, the body will not be healthy. When the colon becomes clogged with toxins, these poisons are reabsorbed into the bloodstream, which pollutes the cells. The colon is hindered in its ability to absorb nutrients and water efficiently when an abundance of toxins are present. Bloating and gas develops.

Although the idea of a daily enema as part of the healing process may not seem pleasant, it is of vital importance and will bring the reward of protecting the body from dangerous pathogens trapped within the colon and speed the healing process. The ancient Egyptians practiced enemas as part of their method of healing the sick.

It was important for me to remember that as the result of taking the herbal germ cleanse, toxins present in my body would very quickly be released into my intestinal tract. The colon quickly fills with ammonia, toxic gases, fungi, and bowel bacteria. I learned from Dr. Clark that the faster these harmful toxins in the colon are removed, the faster the body will heal. Dr. Clark says that not doing at least a daily enema will be detrimental to health when taking an herbal germ cleanse, and even more so when taking an herbal germ cleanse while battling a terminal illness. No matter what the illness, mild or severe, a person who is constipated will experience a slowed recovery, nausea and physical weakness as the result of toxins trapped in the colon.

I learned that usually a cancerous tumor does not kill the body unless its rapid growth impedes the function of another organ; rather, the toxins, specifically the bacteria produced by the malignant tumor, kill the body. This served as a motivation for me to be diligent in carrying out the task of a daily enema during the 18 day healing process. If I had just flatly refused to do enemas, I could have scheduled colonics during the healing process.

The colon wall contains a large number of small finger-like parts which protrude from the inner wall of the small intestine. These are referred to as villi. The body absorbs nutrients through villi. The villi lose their ability to efficiently absorb nutrients when fecal matter and mucus are compressed upon the colon wall. This condition also serves to create chronic constipation. The end result is poor absorption, meaning although nutritious food may be eaten, the body is unable to efficiently absorb the nutrients, creating a gradual breakdown in health.

In combination with the necessary enemas, I learned the way to quickly remove this waste from my colon was to use a good colon cleanse product, if necessary; stay hydrated with alkaline water and medicinal teas; eat a healthy diet; and to get some exercise daily. It is important to take ground flax seed, chia seed or Psyllium with your food, a teaspoon or more at a time, three times a day. Fiber Smart by Renew Life contains probiotics which help to rebuild the body, enabling the body to fight disease. Fiber helps to strengthen and tone the colon muscles as well as absorbing or gathering the toxins in the digestive tract, allowing the toxins to quickly pass out of the body.

Preparing for an Enema

For the sake of convenience, I used a disposable Fleet enema bottle or its generic version. I found this much easier than juggling an enema bag around. This can be purchased at the grocery store or pharmacy very inexpensively, or use a regular enema bag. Never use anyone else's equipment for this. Enema equipment can often be purchased at better health food stores, and there is a large variety of this type of equipment which may be purchased online on my website. Avoid using latex equipment.

I learned from reading Dr. Clark's writings that when ready to use the enema, if choosing to use the suggested disposable Fleet enema, be sure and pour the contents of the disposable enema down the drain and rinse it thoroughly. This is important because the ingredients in the commercial product may be toxic. Be sure and clean off the petroleum lubricant on the nozzle, as well, and instead apply olive oil or Miracle II Neutralizer Gel as a lubricant.

Fill the enema bottle with very warm water. Very warm water is much easier to hold in the bowel than cold water. Administer the enema to cleanse the bowel. Rinse the bottle with some hot water and Miracle II Soap.

Now prepare either one to four teaspoons of black walnut hull extra strength to one quart of very warm distilled water or add 1/8 ounce of Miracle II Soap and two ounces of Miracle II Neutralizer in a quart of warm distilled water; then refill the bottle or the enema bag. I prefer using the Miracle II products, but the black walnut is a good way to cleanse also.

Administer the enema until you reach the point where you are able to comfortably hold the liquid for 10 to 15 minutes. Holding the enema for 10 to 15 minutes helps to insure the maximum amount of toxins is released during the one procedure, according to Dr. Clark. Holding the enema any longer can allow the toxins to be reintroduced into the bloodstream. Practice will make perfect on this one.

Another reason it is so important to have enemas while you take an anti-cancer herbal cleanse is a portion of the colon near the rectum may balloon out into a pocket as the result of past constipation. This is actually a very typical condition. This pocket is referred to as a diverticulum. The pocket is just a few inches from the anus, so it is easily accessed by an enema. The diverticulum walls are weak from constant overstretching, but the diverticulum will shrink down and may even disappear after a few weeks of daily cleansing.

The harmful germs, bacteria and fungi will escape being killed if they are hidden in the diverticulum. Bowel health can only be restored by removing all of the toxins.

A daily enema is just as important as taking the herbal products. When the germs die as the result of the herbal germ cleanse, there is a release of extremely toxic bacteria, and the sooner this bacterium is removed, the better the body will feel. When I was able, I took two enemas a day.

If I experienced constipation, I took an herbal laxative. I found Nature's Sunshine products were helpful in cleansing the bowel.

Items Needed For an Enema

1. Black walnut extra strength tincture or Miracle II Soap (the plain not the moisturizing soap) and Neutralizer.
2. Two (Fleet) disposable enema bottles per enema. Avoid using any latex enema products, as latex is toxic to the body!
3. Olive oil or Miracle II Neutralizer Gel to lubricate the nozzle
4. Miracle II Soap and very warm water
5. Clean towels
6. A large plastic garbage bag to be used as a cover for the floor
7. A paper plate to set used equipment on
8. Dr. Clark's hand sanitizer for cleanup. This can be purchased from my website for around $5 per bottle. Do not use a hand sanitizer containing any isopropyl alcohol, as you will not get well if you are continually exposed to isopropyl alcohol. It is permissible to use products containing ethyl alcohol.
9. A scrubbing brush for cleaning under the fingernails, and there is always the option of using disposable gloves.

When ready to take the enema, place the clean plastic garbage bag on the bathroom floor, and place a large towel over the bag. Lie down on the towel on your left side, administer the enema, and hold it for 10 to 15 minutes.

If there is a feeling of being unable to hold any more of the enema water or cramping, stop the enema, take some deep breaths, and roll from side to side. It is better to start out holding small amounts for at least 10 minutes than to be unable to retain the enema for a full 10 minutes. It may be easier to retain the enema water if taken on the knees with the face down and the rear end up in the air. After becoming more practiced at administering the enema, put a garbage bag and towel on a bed, and rest more comfortably.

Obviously, if caring for someone who is very ill, the enema may have to be given while the person lies in bed as the result of being too weak to get up. Following through with one enema, and the use of a bedpan may detox the system enough to enable them to get up from the bed. Wear a disposable mask with a plastic shield and gloves as protection when administering an enema to someone else.

It is very important to be extremely careful to clean up after an enema. The spread of bacteria has the potential of impeding or preventing healing. Always use Lugol's hand sanitizer, Germaclenz from the North American Herb & Spice Company or a similar product after cleanup.

Coffee Enemas

The next step is said to assist in detoxification of the liver. Along with drinking an adequate amount of water to hydrate the body, an organic coffee enema will help detox the liver by opening the bile ducts and allowing the toxins to be released. Do not omit this step, as this will tremendously aid in recovery.

The following is the recipe for coffee enemas: boil ¾ cup of ground organic coffee with one quart of spring or distilled water for 15 minutes. Wilson coffee is a brand made exclusively for coffee enemas. Strain out the grounds, and separate into four cups for refrigeration. The ratio is one cup of coffee to three cups of water, heated to slightly warmer than body temperature when you get ready to administer the enema. If the caffeine in this coffee gives you the jitters, add some chamomile tea to the enema solution.

1. Take the enema following a bowel movement, or first empty your colon with a warm water enema rather than waiting for nature to take its course.
2. If there is an intestinal gas problem, do some floor exercises prior to administering an enema in an effort to expel the gas.
3. Lie on the left side while administering the enema.
4. The enema may lower blood sugar. If you experience this, make it a practice of eating something before taking the enema.
5. If nothing comes out after holding the enema for 10 minutes, it is most likely because of dehydration. You need to drink more water. NOTE: It is very important to not exceed three weeks of coffee enemas; abuse of coffee enemas can cause you to become anemic!

Colonic Hydrotherapy

Colonic hydrotherapy is a gentle, extended way of cleansing the colon with a gentle infusion of filtered, temperature-controlled water into the colon. A disposable speculum allows warm water to travel through approximately five feet of the large intestines, softening and loosening waste and debris. When the urge to evacuate grows stronger, the water is then safely eliminated along with waste and toxins by just a flip of a switch, leaving the colon through a clear tube connected to the device. The system is fully enclosed, so there is no mess or odor. This process assists the natural muscle contraction called peristalsis, the muscle contraction which moves the waste through the colon.

Any colonic hydrotherapist will tell you laxatives inflame and irritate the colon, draining the body of water, essential minerals and physical energy. Enemas clean only the lower portion of the bowel, leaving a large section of the colon full of toxic waste. The most efficient measure taken to eliminate toxins in the colon is colonic hydrotherapy. The colonic hydrotherapy cleanses all of the way to the sigmoid colon. It is not a cure for an illness or disease, but it relieves the body of toxins, allowing the healing process to begin. Remember, eliminate the toxic burden and the body can heal! Doctors who practice alternative medicine are big proponents of colonic hydrotherapy and send their patients by the droves for this procedure. They realize that when toxins are removed from the colon, their patients' health will improve.

An effective cleansing program involves a series of these infusions, and the number will vary for each person. An initial series of three treatments within a ten-day period is recommended. When combined with a healthy diet and exercise, the colonic aids in detoxifying, rebuilding, and rejuvenating the body. I understand many Hollywood stars have colonic hydrotherapy before walking the red carpet, as it flattens the belly and makes the skin glow.

There are conditions when a colonic is not recommended, such as kidney cancer. My colonic hydrotherapist, a seasoned veteran in a number of alternative medicine treatments, related to me some of the other contra-indications are completely unfounded as it is such a gentle procedure.

However, she agreed a person with kidney cancer should not have colonic hydrotherapy.

A colonic has a cleansing effect on more than just the colon itself. A colonic hydrates the body and opens the lymphatic system, allowing the lymphatics to properly drain.

In addition to being a valuable tool for cleansing the colon of blocked fecal matter, a colonic aids in cleansing germs, bacteria, mucus and fungus from the colon. This can aid in eliminating chronic headaches, backaches, constipation, diarrhea, abdominal gas and bloating, skin problems, menstrual problems, infertility, fatigue, depression, or anxiety—symptoms which indicate the colon is in need of a cleanse. I have read of women who were unable to conceive and quickly became pregnant following a series of colonics, as the bulky presence of impacted fecal material can very easily hinder a woman's ability to conceive.

When I was ill, I knew having a colonic was the right choice, but I dreaded the first visit. My anxious feelings proved to be completely unwarranted, though, as it was a gentle procedure and not at all uncomfortable.

CHAPTER 22

Food Grade Hydrogen Peroxide Restoring My Health for Just Pennies a Day

Being confident of this very thing, that he
who has begun a good work in you will be
faithful to perform it…—Philippians 2:6

I found that 35% food grade hydrogen peroxide (H202) is an amazing product that enabled me to completely restore my health for just pennies a day. H202 is naturally produced in nature, and is commonly used in the food industry to sterilize containers before they are filled with food products. Hearing this and reading much more about the many experiences of others using this natural remedy, I felt confident about "taking a leap of faith" and trying it out for myself.

Though I found treating with H202 is effective and inexpensive, I also learned it requires discipline. If for some reason I decided to stop treating with H202, I learned I should not stop the treatment abruptly, but rather gradually decrease the dosage.

A leading proponent of the usefulness of H202 in the battle against cancer is Dr. William Campbell Douglass, M.D., who wrote a book entitled *Hydrogen Peroxide-Medical Miracle*. If I were facing lung cancer, I would purchase his book. The book is available on my website for less than $15.00, www.ibeatcancers.com.

155

Listed below are some of the diseases which have favorably responded to oxygen therapy, according to Dr. David G. Williams, author of *"Secrets of Life Extension: 10 Simple All-Natural Steps to Achieving Your Natural Lifespan."* Dr. Williams is an adamant and seasoned proponent of treating with H202 as a means to successfully fight disease and restore health:

Allergies
Altitude Sickness
Alzheimer's
Anemia
Arrhythmia
Asthma
Bacterial Infections
Bronchitis
Cancer
Candida/Chronic Yeast Infection
Cardiovascular Disease
Cerebral Vascular Disease
Chronic Pain
Diabetes Type II
Diabetic Gangrene
Diabetic Retinopathy,
Digestion Problems
Epstein-Barr virus
Emphysema
Food Allergies
Fungal Infections
Gingivitis
Headaches
Hepatitis C
Herpes Simplex
Herpes Zoster
HIV Infection
Influenza
Insect Bites
Liver Cirrhosis

Lupus
Multiple Sclerosis
Parasitic Infections
Parkinson's Disease
Periodontal Disease
Prostatitis
Rheumatoid Arthritis
Sinusitis
Shingles
Sore throats
Viral infections
Warts

I learned the body actually produces H202 to fight infection, and that H202 must be present for our immune system to function properly. White blood cells are known as Leukocytes. A sub-class of Leukocytes called Neutrophils produce H202 as the first line of defense against toxins, parasites, bacteria, viruses and yeast. As we age, the body's ability to naturally produce H202 slows, and this plays a part in why people are more likely to develop cancer and heart disease as they age. Chemotherapy and radiation stimulate the Neutrophils into producing H202. Many doctors who practice alternative medicine administer H202 IV infusions to heal various conditions which are considered incurable by conventional medicine. Supplementing with H202 naturally aids the body in rebuilding the immune system.

I realized I could safely use H202, but I learned that there were definitely easy-to-follow, but very important rules, that I must observe if I were going to use it without harming my body.

WHAT I LEARNED ABOUT
USING 35% FOOD GRADE H202

1. 35% H202 comes with a WARNING: Hydrogen peroxide is caustic in high concentrations and should be kept out of reach of children, as even swallowing one teaspoon of undiluted 35% H202 can be fatal.

2. 35% H202 is commonly used in the production of foods, such as cheese, eggs and whey-containing products, as H202 eliminates and prevents bacteria. It is also sprayed on the foil lining of aseptic packages containing fruit juices.

3. 35% H202 is the only grade of hydrogen peroxide recommended for internal use; the hydrogen peroxide sold at the local drug store contains stabilizers and is unfit for human consumption.

4. 35% H202 should be refrigerated and keeping it in a freezer is the optimum way of storage, as this prevents the breakdown of its potency.

5. 35% H202 should be handled with rubber gloves as it will bleach skin.

6. One of the most convenient methods of dispensing 35%H202 is filling a small bottle that has an eye dropper with H202. I store the small bottle in the refrigerator and store the larger container in my freezer.

7. 35% H202 should be used with either **distilled** water, vegetable or fruit juice, milk or even aloe vera juice or gel. At first I drank it with distilled water, but as the dosage increased, I found it was easier to drink it in 6 ounces of juice (V-8 is my favorite) or with 6 ounces of almond milk. When I drank it with water, I used 12 ounces of water.

8. 35% H202 dosages must be very gradually increased, and I have included a chart I followed in this chapter.

9. 35% H202 must only be taken on an empty stomach, at least 3 hours after a meal, and that I should not eat anything for 1 hour after taking H202.

10. 35% H202 can cause nausea, and that decreasing the next dosage by one drop would help decrease nausea.

11. Taking 4 or 5 lecithin capsules with each dose of 35% H202 helped eliminate nausea, as did ginger root capsules.

12. Taking 2 or 3 capsules of Dr. Clark's wild source rose hip vitamin C, 550 mg. and 2 capsules of Dr. Clark's betaine hydrochloride one hour following a dose of 35% H202 would also aid in relieving any nausea.

13. I learned that I should never abruptly stop using H202, but rather gradually taper off its use. This is extremely important, as abruptly

stopping can trigger an outbreak of any type of virus suppressed by the immune system.

14. I learned to avoid eating foods containing vinegar while treating with H202, i.e., salad dressing or pickled vegetables. If I mistakenly ate anything with vinegar, I immediately felt a puckering discomfort in the palate, but no severe symptoms. I also learned that it was extremely important to avoid drinking canned beverages of any sort while treating with H202. This is because of the heavy metals present in canned beverages.

15. I learned that if I planned on taking high doses of H202 for a period longer than 30 days, it was extremely important for me to take the following anti-oxidant supplements to protect my healthy cells from oxidative stress. The following list was provided in a booklet entitled *"Hydrogen Peroxide Therapy,"* by Conrad LeBeau. I learned it was important to take these supplements one hour following a dose of H202.

RECOMMENDED ANTI-OXIDANTS

a. Pycnogenol – 30 mg. 3 to 5 times a day; pycnogenol is an herbal supplement that is regarded for its anti-oxidant properties. It is used for battling free radicals within the body to prevent aging and circulation issues.

b. Vitamin A - 10,000 to 25,000 i.u. daily

c. Beta-carotene – 50 to 100 mg. daily

d. Vitamin C – 1,000 to 5,000 mg. daily

e. Vitamin E – 400 i.u. once or twice a day

f. Selenium – 50 mg. 3 times a day

Dr. Williams, author of *"Secrets of Life Extension: 10 Simple All-Natural Steps to Achieving Your Natural Lifespan,"* states that this outlined program is only a suggestion, but it is based on years of experience, and reports from thousands of users. According to Dr. Williams, those who choose to go at a slower pace can expect to progress more slowly, but that certainly is an option. The program is not carved in stone, and he says to keep in mind that it can be adapted to fit individual needs. Dr. Williams **warns that**

individuals who have had transplants should not undertake an H2O2 program. H2O2 stimulates the immune system and could possibly cause a rejection of the organ.

Day #/Number of Drops/ Times Per Day

1 - 3 / 3
2 - 4 / 3
3 - 5 / 3
4 - 6 / 3
5 - 7 / 3
6 - 8 / 3
7 - 9 / 3
8 - 10 / 3
9 - 12 / 3
10 - 14 / 3
11 - 16 / 3
12 - 18 / 3
13 - 20 / 3
14 - 22 / 3
15 - 24 / 3
16 - 25 / 3
17 - 25 /3
18 - 25 /3
19 - 25 /3
20 - 25 /3
21 – 25/3

Maintenance Dosage

According to Dr. Williams, it is perfectly fine to continue taking H2O2 three times a day in small doses, i.e., 3 to 7 drops, which is how I take it. In most situations after the above 21 day program, the amount of H2O2 should be tapered off gradually as follows:

25 drops once every other day for 1 week;
25 drops once every third day for 2 weeks;

25 drops once every fourth day for 3 weeks:

MY PERSONAL EXPERIENCE WITH
35 % FOOD GRADE H202

After purchasing 35% Food Grade Hydrogen Peroxide, I stored it away in the refrigerator, not knowing exactly where to begin. After a few months passed, I happened upon some information which made some impressive claims regarding the usefulness of H202; this prompted me to do an intense Internet search. What I read in the Internet search was nothing short of amazing. There was lots of information available on the Internet, and I even located a free and extremely informative e-book entitled *"The Truth about Food Grade Hydrogen Peroxide."*

Initially, I felt a bit apprehensive about getting started because 35% H202 came with some serious warnings on handling and storage, but I carefully read the directions and pressed on. I was amazed by how quickly my body responded to its use.

I began with 2 drops, 3 times a day and very slowly moved up to the higher doses. At higher doses, I experienced nausea, but found taking lecithin and ginger when I took H202, and vitamin C, along with betaine hydrochloride an hour after taking H202, really helped to relieve the nausea. Once in a while I experienced a slight feeling of nausea, but it was not unbearable. I was able to continue with my day-to-day life activities, such as working out at the gym. I did read a blog in which several individuals experienced no nausea at all while treating with H202.

The requirement of taking a dose of H202 on an empty stomach meant taking a dose first thing in the morning and waiting 1 hour before eating. After eating, I then had to wait 3 hours before having another dose, and, of course, that also meant waiting 1 hour before eating again. This wasn't always convenient, but I pressed on with the use of H202 as I wanted to get completely well. I went at a much slower pace and did not go past 16 drops, 3 times a day.

I noticed any plaque that had been on my teeth came off in shards when I flossed my teeth; my teeth now felt as though I had just had them cleaned. For a number of years, I have had my teeth cleaned every 3 months, at my dental hygienist's suggestion, because I had a problem with accumulating a lot of plaque on my lower front teeth due to wearing a mouth guard at night. I can now see why H2O2 is reportedly so effective in eliminating heart disease, as it eliminates a build-up of plaque.

Earlier I mentioned how I had been able to shrink the baseball-sized tumor in my breast to less than the size of a small grain of rice. Since I still had this tiny linear tumor, I was forced to restrict my diet, avoid eating any plant in the allium family, and avoid non-organic meats and dairy because of their estrogen content. I also strictly avoided grains, fruit and sugars, faithfully adhering to a ketogenic diet.

Previous to treating with H2O2, whenever I ate anything from the "offending" food groups, the area in my breast where the tumor was located would sometimes feel "itchy." Occasionally, I would experience twinges of pain and my breast would show signs of inflammation. I was in a continual battle with my health, but I pressed on, knowing I had no alternative. Each time I faced signs of inflammation in my breast, which I considered a "crisis," I would resolve to do better, which meant I would stay with my ketogenic diet and faithfully take supplements. Around day 3 of treating with H2O2, I no longer experienced any signs of breast cancer, no feeling of itchiness, no twinges of pain or any inflammation, regardless of what I ate. Although, I continued to avoid non-organic meats and dairy at home, I was now free to dine out at a restaurant or eat at a friend's house without being restricted in my diet.

Not only did I no longer suffer any symptoms with my breast regardless of what I ate, but I no longer required the use of any cancer remedies. I gradually reduced the amount of H2O2 I was using and decided to continue drinking 3 to 7 drops, 2 or 3 times a day, on a daily basis. I learned it was perfectly fine for me to continue on with this course of treatment and that not only would it not hurt my health, but it would serve to keep me disease free.

Dr. Williams suggested that if a person is unable to tolerate treating with higher dosages of H2O2 or are not achieving their desired results, they should seek out a physician who administers H2O2 intravenously, which is a more effective treatment. He recommended searching for a physician who administers chelation therapy, as they would be familiar with H2O2 IV treatment.

Treating with H2O2 intravenously has been safely used for over 100 years successfully. In fact, Dr. Williams stated that a doctor used it during the influenza epidemic of World War I with great results and saved many lives. To be safe, this treatment is not used in pregnancy, chronic granulomatous diseases, and hemolytic anemia. It may cause side-effects associated with any intravenous therapy such as vasculitis, infusion site pain, and bruising. It may also cause a Herxheimer reaction from dying microorganisms, which may include flu-like symptoms, such as headache, fatigue, grouchiness, insomnia, nausea and muscle pain. These symptoms are temporary and represent the body detoxifying and clearing infections and toxins. The symptom that I was most aware when I began using H202 was hot flashes, just for a few days though. I learned that this was an indication of the H202 cleansing my body of cancerous cells.

Making and Using 3% Solutions of H202

A 3% solution can be made quite easily by first pouring 1 ounce of 35% H202 into a pint jar. To this add 11 ounces of distilled water. This will make 12 ounces of 3% H202. 3% H202 has a variety of medicinal uses.

1. It can be used full strength as a mouthwash (avoid swallowing) or mixed with baking soda for toothpaste.
2. It can be used full strength as a foot bath for athlete's foot. (Diabetics have found relief from circulation problems by soaking their feet in 1 pint of 3% peroxide mixed with 1 gallon of warm, non-chlorinated water for 30 minutes nightly.)
3. A tablespoon added to 1 cup of non-chlorinated water can be used as a nasal spray. Depending on the degree of sinus involvement, one will have to adjust the amount of peroxide used. The author of this article claimed they had seen some who can use it at the full 3% strength (I would never try that) and others who had difficulty with using a few drops mixed with a cup of water.
4. 3% H202 can be added to a pet's drinking water at the rate of 1 ounce per quart of non-chlorinated water.

According to Dr. Williams, there are a number of companies who make products using H202. He warns that you'll end up paying a small fortune with these products and at the very best you will achieve the same results you can get for pennies a day by using H202.

CHAPTER 23

Avoiding Foods with Mold

And God said, Behold, I have given you every herb
bearing seed, which is upon the face of all the earth,
and every tree, in the which is the fruit of a tree yielding
seed; to you it shall be for meat.—Genesis1:29

Almost everyone likes apples and has heard the old adage, "An apple a day keeps the doctor away." Well, this is true. The fiber in an apple will help keep the colon moving in the right direction and thus prevent a buildup of bacteria and fungus due to constipation.

However, I have learned that fruit can harbor mold. What looks like a little brown spot on an apple is actually mold, also called mycotoxins. Dr. Clark claimed that eating mold will cause a sudden drop in the immune system and allow viruses suppressed by our own immune system to surface once again.

Fruit is most certainly good for us, but it must be carefully examined. I learned that while I battled cancer I needed to avoid all fruit. I also learned that after recovering from the disease, I need to only eat fruit in its prime condition.

Berries may be eaten, but look them over very carefully before purchasing them, as they mold very easily. The skin is thin on berries, and berries have a lot of nooks and crannies that can easily hold undesirable pesticide residue; for this reason, it is best to eat organic berries. You can purchase frozen organic berries year round.

Since ascorbic acid discourages mold, Dr. Clark recommended putting a pinch of vitamin C, ascorbic acid, into a fruit dish we are about to eat. She also recommended a pinch of vitamin C be added to our homemade jams and jellies every time we open the jar to take a portion out, as these jars can be a great breeding ground for mold. Commercial jams and jellies are not a good choice because of mold, but there is the option of eating them with a pinch of vitamin C. However, according to Dr. Clark, during the healing process, commercially prepared grape jelly and jam should be avoided altogether, as they likely harbor mold.

According to Dr. Clark, those who suffer with cancer of the brain should avoid all fruit and berries, as an allergy can exist and trigger this type of cancer.

Other foods which commonly harbor mold are nuts and nut butters. Additionally, a pinch of vitamin C should be sprinkled inside the jar of nut butter before closing and storing in the refrigerator. This discourages the presence of mold.

Commercial bread stored in plastic also regularly contains mold; better to choose homemade bread made with unbleached flour, or second best, bakery bread which is not stored in plastic.

I purchase sour dough millet bread from the health food store for my husband. This bread, which contains no yeast, is stored in the freezer. I keep it in the freezer at home, too, and just take out the amount he is going to eat for a meal. Of course, while you are going through the healing process, avoid grains. You may eat in moderation products made with coconut flour and almond flour.

Potatoes and bulk grains can also contain mold, so they should be carefully examined and boiled with salt so the boiling point is raised. The best choice following your complete recovery is to eat wild rice and the best potatoes to select are red potatoes. Dr. Clark recommended eating white rice, rather than brown because of the presence of mold in brown rice.

Beer contains mold, and wine is made using fungus. These beverages are not acceptable choices for someone who has cancer or suffered with it previously.

High fructose corn syrup is inexpensive and plentiful, which makes it a popular sweetener for manufacturers. Unfortunately, high fructose corn syrup is a product which contains mercury, causes leaky gut and fosters mold in the body, feeds candida, making it particularly dangerous for anyone with a weakened immune system. I have learned in all of my research that high fructose corn syrup promotes disease in the body, and eating high fructose corn syrup is so unnecessary, as there are quality substitutes that do not ruin good health, i.e., stevia and xylitol.

A macrobiotic diet removes mycotoxins from the diet. For that reason, people are very often healed of cancer when they adopt the macrobiotic lifestyle.

I believe the reason I have been so successful in combatting the disease of cancer is the result of my diet change. Regardless of the time of year or the occasion, I remain faithful to a ketogenic diet. There are so many wonderful books which offer ketogenic recipes, such as the ones penned by Doug Kauffman; there are also the wonderful Paleo Diet cookbooks; and these can be purchased online from www.ibeatcancers.com.

CHAPTER 24

Acid-Forming Sources to Avoid

Every word of God is pure; he is a shield to them
that put their trust in him.—Proverbs 30:5

I learned that in order for my body to heal speedily, the pH of my saliva should test from 7.36 to 7.44. When the body is acidic, disease is permitted to flourish. The most important thing I learned while on the 18-day herbal germ cleanse was how to *stop feeding* the cancer by eating the wrong foods. The following is a list of highly acidic substances, which should be avoided in order to reach and maintain good health:

1. Coffee: other than using coffee for enemas
2. Tobacco: if you use tobacco, you will not get well. Avoid being around tobacco smoke altogether, as it causes tumor growth.
3. Alcoholic beverages in all forms
4. Black tea
5. Carbonated beverages, even the ones without sugar or health food store sodas.
6. White refined sugars, table sugar, artificial sugars, honey, maple syrup, agave and high fructose corn syrup. Avoid eating any sweets.
7. Stress, worry, fear, and anxiety
8. Commercial cleaners and chlorine

Are all acids bad? Absolutely not! The human body has been designed to work best with a healthy balance of good acids and good alkalines that keep each other in check.

Examples of acids that are healthy and very necessary to good health are essential fatty acids—EFAs—nuts, seeds, fish, and avocados. I learned the body requires a small amount of fat in order to properly absorb nutrients.

CHAPTER 25

Foods & Substances to Avoid While Battling Cancer

Touch not; taste not; handle not.—Colossians 2:21

When I learned what foods I was eating which actually encouraged the presence of cancer-causing germs, I was nothing short of astonished, as these were foods I ate nearly every day with the assumption they were keeping me healthy. I avoided these foods for years until I found a solution, which I outline in Chapter 22. The foods I avoided are vegetables in the allium family.

These foods are good for you unless you have developed cancer. The cancer-causing germ, which is killed by the herbal germ cleanse, thrives on the alkylating agents found in plants in the allium family. I later learned that taking 35% food grade hydrogen peroxide on a daily basis would allow me to safely eat anything I wanted to, but while doing the germ cleanse, avoid the vegetables in the allium family listed below.

Carefully check the list of ingredients in all processed foods and condiments in order to prevent ingesting any of the following:

- Onions
- Garlic
- Leeks
- Chives
- Shallots

- Asparagus
- Mustard

The following is a list of foods which should be avoided during the healing process. Some contain food allergens which weaken the immune system; and some contain estrogen, a substance which is deadly to one who suffers with hormonal cancer. Even though many of these foods contain nutritional value, they should be avoided by anyone battling cancer:

Also included in this list are some over-the-counter medications associated with the disease of cancer or that burden the liver, causing health to weaken:

- Alfalfa sprouts (A strong risk of bacteria)
- Acetaminophen (Burdens the liver)
- Aspirin (Causes bleeding and leads to pain; also associated with some cancers, i.e., leukemia)
- Beans, dried peas, lentils, and garbanzo beans (You may eat black beans and lentils after you recover.)
- Beef (Avoid unless it is organic, grass-fed beef)
- Black tea (Herbal teas are encouraged, as they have properties that heal the body.)
- Cabbage (Avoid with bone cancer)
- Carrots (Avoid with liver cancer)
- Cashews, peanuts and pistachios (Instead choose raw seeds and raw nuts, such as walnuts, pecans, pine nuts, Brazil nuts, sunflower seeds, pumpkin seeds, hemp hearts, etc., purchased from the refrigerated section of the health food store.)
- Chicken and eggs when non-organic (Just as with pork, non-organic chicken and eggs are often raised in conditions which harbor bacteria. To combat the bacterial problems, as well as increasing their weight at the market, chickens are fed antibiotics and estrogen. These substances are then passed onto the consumer. If a person eats these foods day in and day out, year after year, they are accumulating these toxins. Sooner or later, these toxins will result in disease in the body. Chicken packaged with a label stating it is raised without hormones or antibiotics is permitted.

Eggs are associated with a lot of bacteria. It is important to wash the eggshell before cracking it open for use.)

- Cinnamon (Contains an acid that can lead to food allergy; associated with bladder cancer) Use coriander instead.
- Coffee (In order for the body to heal, the bloodstream must be alkaline. There are several cancers associated with caffeine: brain, spine, optic nerve and esophageal cancers. Organo Gold makes an alkaline coffee that I love; my favorite is King of Coffees; find this at www.ibeatcancers.com. Try drinking Black Chaga or White Chaga in place of coffee, also on my website. Chaga makes the body strong. A great beverage for a person in a weakened state.)
- Corn (Connected with many cancers, as well as mold, in the body.)
- Non-organic dairy products (The dairy products should be raw if at all possible; locate a source through RealMilk.com. Be vigilant about sterilizing dairy. Completely avoid dairy in the case of cancer of the nipple and milk ducts, as this cancer is due to an allergic reaction to the phenylalanine contained in dairy products. Kidney cancer is associated with a casein allergy (cheese). Dairy products contain great nutrition, but they can also slow peristalsis (digestion) and create mucus within the body; for this reason, they may slow the healing process. I learned if a person is lactose intolerant, it is best to avoid dairy.)
- Fennel is high in phytoestrogens and should be avoided in the case of estrogenic cancer
- Fried foods (Carcinogenic, meaning cancer causing)
- Fruit (Avoid all fruit during the healing process.)
- GMO (Avoid genetically modified foods (GMO), as they increase the likelihood of the body developing tumors as well as allergies.)
- Grain (Enriched or bleached flour, grains are treated with chlorine and preservatives for a long shelf life and contain gallic acid, a link to pancreatic cancer, according to Dr. Hulda Clark's book *The Cure & Prevention of all Cancers*.) A better choice is to begin eating foods made with almond flour and coconut flour.
- Grilled or barbequed meats cooked with propane gas or charcoal grilled, even broiled meats (Foods cooked in this manner are carcinogenic and will cause an infection in the lower bowel,

indicated by stool which is no wider than one inch wide. Best to eat slowly cooked meats when you are sick. I learned that treating with 35% food grade hydrogen peroxide will heal this type of infection in the lower bowel.)

- High fructose corn syrup (High fructose corn syrup promotes dental decay, leaky gut, produces anxiety in children and aches and pains in adults and destroys health! Shame on greedy manufacturers for using this as a sweetener.)
- Honey (Avoid completely as a cancer patient. Dr. Clark claimed that cancer patients are allergic to honey.)
- Ibuprofen (Burdens the liver)
- Lunch meats and hot dogs (Meats are sold by the pound; so in order to increase their profit margin, farmers have employed the use of hormones and antibiotics, as well as other pharmaceutical drugs to increase the weight of livestock. Even the expensive so-called "quality luncheon meats" contain harmful estrogens. Remember, if it does not say organic, it is not organic, even though the manufacturer may boast that their product has no chemicals.)
- Maple syrup
- Molasses
- MSG also known as carrageen, an ingredient frequently found in dairy products (Toxic to the body and is associated with cancer of the tongue)
- Non-organic meats (A heavy source of dangerous growth hormones, and antibiotics)
- Oats (Oats are a grain, of course, but I wanted to mention them exclusively as they are associated with "healthy eating." Dr. Clark said oats feed the cancer-causing germ that is associated with liver cancer)
- Oils - The following new-fangled [man-made] fats can cause cancer, heart disease, immune system dysfunction, sterility, learning disabilities, growth problems and osteoporosis:
All hydrogenated oils, soy, corn, safflower oil, cottonseed oil, canola oil, all fats heated to very high temperatures in processing and frying.
- Oranges, tangerines (Avoid with throat cancer)

- Peppers (Except jalapeno seeds)
- Pork (As the result of modern farming methods, this meat contains antibiotics and bacteria which are resistant to drugs or entire classes of drugs. What this means to you is if you contract a bacterial infection as the result of eating these pork products, a treating physician would have to prescribe a more powerful antibiotic as a curative measure; antibiotics weaken the immune system. Pork is frequently associated with urinary tract infections and foodborne illnesses. It is particularly dangerous to feed pork to children, the elderly, and the infirm. Whenever we ingest the meat of a diseased animal, we are also ingesting the disease it suffered with; eating this diseased flesh is harmful to our health. Personally, I would not eat even organic pork. I read that after consuming a meal of pork, you can test positive in a test for cancer for up to a week.)
- Potatoes (Undercooked or fried, they are especially dangerous to good health. Now that I have recovered my health, I choose organic red potatoes, without the slightest hint of green in the peel, as this is toxic.)
- Raw cruciferous vegetables (Vegetables, such as broccoli, cauliflower, kohlrabi, etc.; eating these vegetables lightly steamed is highly recommended, as this breaks down the cell wall of the plant and does not interfere with iodine absorption. Cruciferous vegetables draw harmful estrogens from the body. Whenever dining out, order broccoli or other cruciferous vegetables to help protect against the bad estrogens in the food you have ordered. The supplement DIM is made from broccoli and cabbage and is an excellent product to take in order to eliminate harmful estrogens in the body.)
- Shrimp (AVOID ALL SHELLFISH) When God told His people to shun shellfish and pork in the dietary laws, He was warning them that these things were harmful to the health of the people He loved.
- Sodium hydrochloride or table salt (This salt is an enemy of the immune system; switch to pink Himalayan salt.)
- Soy products, including soy oil (Soy contains phytoestrogens and promotes estrogen dominance. Soy ingestion is directly related to

diseases of the thyroid and is linked to the early onset of puberty in girls who were fed soy in infant formula. As healthy as it may sound, soy is an estrogen and must be avoided by anyone with hormonal cancer.) Avoid soy sauce, teriyaki sauce and other Oriental food sauces as they also contain yeast and will feed the cancer.

- Sugar feeds the disease of cancer. It is for this reason you must avoid sugar in all forms during the healing process, i.e., maple syrup, honey, high fructose corn syrup, brown sugar, coconut sugar, agave and even stevia. You will not fully recover from cancer if you insist on eating sweeteners. Find another way to reward yourself! A walk in the park, time with friends and taking up a new hobby can all be forms of enjoyment!

- Sugar substitutes (Splenda or NutraSweet must be avoided. These aspartame sweeteners break down the immune system by destroying beneficial intestinal micro flora and allow pathogenic bacteria to flourish in the gut. They gradually weaken the body by reducing nutrient absorption, resulting in a depletion of Vitamin K2, the vitamin which affects clotting, which then leads to arterial calcification and connective tissue disorders as well as raising insulin levels in the body. Artificial sweeteners are associated with an increased risk of irritability, mood swings, obesity, cancer, type II diabetes and cardiovascular disease. Many cancers are directly related to artificial sweeteners, i.e., brain cancer. Artificial sweeteners are also associated with hair loss.)

- Uncooked or undercooked squash or pumpkin

- Vinegar (Those with prostate or colon cancer should especially avoid ingesting vinegar during the healing process.)

An excellent anti-cancer diet to follow is Doug Kauffman's Phase One Diet, an antifungal diet which can be easily located on an Internet search. Doug Kauffman's television program, Know the Cause, features cutting-edge supplements in the battle against disease. He interviews guests who have been healed of cancer by changing their diets and using the supplements he frequently features. You can also watch his programs online. His cookbooks are available on my website, www.ibeatcancers.com.

SECTION 4

No More Cancer

CHAPTER 26

How I Remain Cancer-Free

And you shall know the truth and the truth
shall make you free. —John 8:32 KJV

1. I supplement with 35% food grade hydrogen peroxide, which I
   have outline in Chapter 22.
2. I strictly avoid products which contain even trace amounts of the
   solvent isopropyl alcohol. If a trip to the doctor has necessitated
   the use of isopropyl alcohol, I quickly take measures to detoxify
   using either an ion foot cleanse or a sauna and a few days of all 3
   herbs in the herbal germ cleanse, or 2 ounces 3 times a day of the
   Juice of Wild Oreganol for a few days in a row, as one application
   of isopropyl alcohol can begin the germ cycle all over again. I
   learned I cannot get well or stay well if I continue to use products
   which contain isopropyl alcohol. I now use ethyl alcohol as a
   suitable substitute.
3. I avoid all forms of chlorine. I learned there will not be a full
   recovery from cancer unless chlorine is avoided, as chlorine causes
   estrogen dominance. Overcoming estrogen dominance is one of the
   keys to recovering health when suffering with a hormonal cancer. I
   use a shower head which filters out chlorine, and when I swim in a
   pool, I take MSM which breaks up the chlorine in the bloodstream.
4. I use only natural personal and household products which contain
   no toxic substances. I learned to go natural! I have featured some
   great natural products on <u>www.ibeatcancers.com</u>.

5. I keep my home and garage free of toxic products.

6. I avoid eating foods which sustain the cancer-causing germ's presence, the plants of the allium family and mustard, unless I have taken my daily dose of H202.

7. I eat only fresh meats which have been cooked until they are falling off the bone. I avoid all processed meats and barbequed and grilled meats.

8. I use stainless steel, glass, enamel cookware or cast iron. I avoid using non-stick cookware or a microwave.

9. I practice some form of detoxification on a daily basis.

CHAPTER 27

Simplicity of Life

To appoint unto them that mourn in Zion, to give unto
them beauty for ashes, the oil of joy for mourning, the
garment of praise for the spirit of heaviness; that they
might be called trees of righteousness, the planting of
the Lord, that he might be glorified.—Isaiah 61:3

I learned that in order to recover from disease and walk in health, it was
imperative I make changes in my lifestyle. Otherwise, my health would
continue in a downward spiral. I came to realize the easiest way to make
these changes was to return to the simplicity of life lived long ago.

From reading Dr. Clark's books, I learned the toxins I encountered in
my home environment and the toxins in the foods I ate every day helped
usher me into a place of poor health.

I also realized there were toxins which could not be avoided, the
pollutants of a modern society, but I learned the importance of
detoxification. I learned that when we neglect detoxification, our bodies
eventually are absolutely overwhelmed by toxins that surround us. We
are soaking up pollutants at a far greater rate than our body's built-in
detoxification system can unload them, and it is vitally important to assist
the body in detoxification.

Eventually, as a result of this toxic overload, disease becomes established
in the body. This is what cancer is, an accumulation of toxins, which
creates a weakness in the body, and this weakness creates an environment

for a bacterial infection. Cancer is not a mystery disease that has an unknown etiology or cause.

We accumulate these toxins from what we eat and how the food is grown, packaged and cooked.

Our bodies soak up toxins from unhealthy grooming products, cleaning products we use to maintain our homes, and even our medicinal remedies, both over-the-counter and pharmaceuticals. We collect toxins from what is added to our water supply. Our bodies gather even more toxins from chemicals sprayed into our environments. All of these toxins serve to weaken or dismantle the body's immune system.

What can we do about this? I found the first step we can take is to begin by using genuinely natural hygiene products, products which have a positive effect on the body, rather than the use of hygiene products containing noxious chemicals which generate disease. In order to stop this epidemic of cancer our society is experiencing, we must return to the use of the simple, natural hygiene products used by some of our ancestors.

Over a hundred years ago, grooming and cleaning supplies were products most often formulated at home from natural substances which were not harmful, unlike most of the products available to us today. In this day and age we are bombarded from every direction by companies touting their beauty products and cleaning products, promising miraculous results, but what is the cost to our health when we use these products? We can oftentimes be exposed to dangerous chemicals, dyes and fragrances that create hormonal changes in the body; unsafe solvents; and a multitude of other harmful hormone-disrupting chemicals, which eventually destroy our health.

The medicinal herbal remedies of our ancestors did not come with outrageously dangerous pharmaceutical warnings. The tonics and curative measures they had at their disposal were such things as vinegar, baking soda, herbal teas, herbal poultices or essential oils for all aspects of their lives.

I really enjoyed receiving and wearing gifts of expensive perfume from my husband until I learned that the high-end department store perfumes I loved were chock full of toxins and were most especially harmful to anyone suffering with cancer. I learned I could not expect to get well if I continued to bathe in or in any way apply these toxin-laden products to my body.

When I began to learn of the magnitude of toxins which were contained in one single bottle of high-end department store perfume, I was horrified.

I want to share a story told to me by a gentleman who lost his wife to a brain tumor. He told me she worked at a high-end department store and during this time she contracted Lyme's disease. Rather than allowing her to stay at home during her illness, the physician provided by her company's insurance required her to work part-time. The department store management reassigned her to work in the fragrance department. He told me she would come home suffering with a migraine headache each day that she worked at the store. His wife pressed on with this awful situation because she was desperate to have health insurance. After just a few months, the headaches became absolutely unbearable and she sought out another physician who ordered a brain scan. The brain scan showed that she was suffering with a fast growing tumor. She lived only a couple of months after the diagnosis. I learned that when a person is already suffering with a disease in their body, they must strictly avoid all environmental toxins. Because their immune system is already in a weakened or declining state, the door is open to further breakdown of their health.

We can and we must choose to make a 180 degree turn away from dangerous products and begin using safe, natural goods. Until we make a commitment to discontinue the use of toxic products, the state of our health and that of our family will be in jeopardy.

The seemingly harmless grooming products polluted with chemicals we apply to our hair and skin every day enter the bloodstream through the skin and lungs. These contaminants take a much heavier toll on the immune system than we may ever wish to contemplate.

Many of us think nothing of placing our bare hands into cleaning products. We do not stop to think that we are absorbing dangerous chemicals into our bodies—chemicals our bodies were not designed to process, chemicals which wreak havoc on the endocrine system and upset the natural rhythm of the body's hormones. These chemicals lodge and collect in the tissue of the body. I learned long-term exposure to these chemicals has a disastrous effect on our health. It is little wonder the disease of cancer is so common in our society and its victims are rapidly increasing in numbers.

A good rule of thumb concerning handling any kind of cleaning substance is this: If you would not ordinarily put this solution into your mouth and swallow it, then by all means, you should not put your bare hands into it. I learned it is important to make a practice of wearing gloves to protect the hands, as the hands are actually portals that allow substances to enter or exit the body through the skin. Likewise, I learned not to walk barefoot in areas where pollutants have been deposited. I have made it a practice of wearing shoes or slippers to protect the bottoms of my feet, as the feet, too, are portals allowing substances to enter/exit the body through the skin.

I learned that commercial dishwasher detergent can leave a toxic residue on dishes. I now use a tablespoon and a half of 20 Mule Team Borax in the dishwasher, along with a teaspoon of citric acid, which can be purchased in bulk—a money-saving change.

I switched to perfume and dye-free laundry detergents. I began to use 20 Mule Team Borax as a laundry booster or laundry detergent and use white vinegar and baking soda or washing soda as a cleaner and laundry booster. I learned that making my own natural laundry soap is a great way to start cleaning up the home environment. The two soap recipes included in this book are a great way to save money on laundry detergent and are easy to make. These recipes come from Wellness Mama, who has great information on her website.

Why switch to natural laundry soap, you ask? Conventional laundry detergent is loaded with chemicals like sulfates, fragrances, phenols, dioxins and more. Many brands contain things like petroleum distillates, which are linked to cancer and lung disease. Fragrances in these detergents are made of a mix of harmful chemicals.

Fortunately, making your own laundry soap is an easy and fast process! You only need three basic ingredients to make either powdered or liquid laundry soap:

- Washing Soda (Arm and Hammer Brand available at most grocery stores)
- Borax (20 Mule Team Borax available at most grocery stores)
- Bar Soap (Dr. Bronner's, Ivory, or other natural, unscented bar soap)

Washing Soda and Borax should be available at your local grocery store on the laundry aisle. Natural bar soaps are in the health, beauty, or organic sections of the store, or online. Adding a couple tablespoons of baking soda helps to freshen the clothing. Borax is a naturally occurring mineral made up of sodium, boron, oxygen, and water. It is an ingredient in most of the natural soaps available now (Seventh Generation, etc.) but you can save money making your own laundry detergent. Washing Soda, sometimes called sodium carbonate or soda ash, is made from common salt and limestone. Dr. Bronner's soaps are made with vegetable castille soap and pure organic oils. Dr. Clark suggested that you avoid Dr. Bronner's peppermint castile soap as she found it contained PCB's.

Natural Laundry Soap Recipe:

1. Grate the bar soap or mix in a food processor until finely ground. Use the soap of your choice. Dr. Bronner's Pure Castille Bar Soap is available in several different natural scents like lavender, tea tree, almond and others.
2. In a large bowl, mix 2 parts washing soda, 2 parts borax and 1 part grated soap. (Add a few teaspoons of baking soda if desired).
3. Store in closed container. If you are using a big enough container, you can skip step 2 and just put all ingredients in storage container or jar and shake.
4. Use 1/8 to 1/4 cup per load of laundry.

Liquid Laundry Soap Recipe:

1. Grate one bar of soap with a cheese grater or food processor.
2. Put grated soap in pan with 2 quarts water and gradually heat, stirring constantly until soap is completely dissolved.
3. Put 4.5 gallons of really hot tap water in a 5-gallon bucket (available for free in bakeries at grocery stores, just ask them) and stir in 1 cup of borax and 1 cup of washing soda until completely dissolved.
4. Pour soap mixture from pan into 5-gallon bucket. Stir well.
5. Cover and leave overnight.

6. Shake or stir until smooth and pour into gallon jugs or other containers.
7. Use 1/2 to 1 cup per load.

If you don't have the time to make your own laundry detergent, purchase Soap Nuts for your laundry needs or use Miracle II Soap without the moisturizer. Miracle II Soap may be used as a window/glass cleaner, car wash, carpet cleaner, spot remover, garden spray, dishwashing soap (not recommended for dishwasher), laundry, oven cleaner, bug spray, dog shampoo, et cetera. Purchase Miracle II products from www. ibeatcancers.com.

Acceptable cleaning products also include hydrogen peroxide, salt, baking soda, lemon juice and the peel of the lemon. Use plain olive oil for furniture polish.

Oregaspray is a North American Herb & Spice product which can be sprayed directly into your air conditioning intake system to kill mold and fungus.

Germaclenz is a North American Herb & Spice product which kills germs on contact when sprayed on surfaces such as steering wheels, telephones, doorknobs, faucet faucets and mattresses, in addition to boosting your immune system when you use it.

Organic Orange TKO is a wonderful nontoxic cleaner and when used in the rinse cycle of the washer, will remove any scent of chlorine products you may have used to remove stains.

There are a myriad of great organic cleaning products, but you must read labels on these products. I found benzene was an ingredient in my organic dishwashing liquid and made the change to Miracle II for a dishwashing liquid. It is actually healthy to place your hands into this soap.

When cleaning with bleach, use NSF-certified bleach, definitely use a mask and gloves, turn on a fan, and ventilate with open windows. Clean your toilets and sink drains once a week with bleach, and store your bleach in the garage or outside.

If you are ill, get someone else to clean with bleach while you sit outside in the open air. It is beneficial to be outdoors every day for as long as you can tolerate, even several times a day. People who spend a lot of time out of doors have longer lifespans. I learned that breathing fresh air is the single most important thing which can be done to strengthen the immune system, and it doesn't cost a dime!

Purchase an ozonator; there are many to choose from on my website at www.ibeatcancers.com. There are ozonators to fit every situation, as well as for your swimming pool and Jacuzzi. An ozonator is an ideal way to purify the air, water and also sterilize freshly cleaned surfaces. Do you live in an apartment and can tell your next door neighbor is smoking? An ozonator is your solution!

During the fifteenth-century outbreak of black plague, a combination of essential oils, known as Thieves' oil, was used by grave robbers to protect them from contracting the same disease which took the lives of the bodies they plundered. This combination of powerful essential oils which protects the body from deadly bacteria is a far cry from the harmful chemical concoctions modern society has come to rely on, i.e., health-robbing hand sanitizers with isopropyl alcohol and aerosol disinfectant sprays which contain harmful hormone-disrupting ingredients.

Essential oils are an important part of the plant's immune system, helping it to fend off attack by yeasts, molds, fungus, viruses, bacteria, and insects. These essential oils offer many excellent alternatives to toxin-laden products our industrialized society has grown accustomed to using on a daily basis—items which pose a very real threat to good health.

Unlike the popular toxic commercial cleaning and personal hygiene products commonly used today, different combinations of essential oils may be safely used in a multitude of ways around the home while also giving the immune system a tremendous boost. These oils contain antibacterial agents which are not harmful to the body, but instead build and strengthen the immune system! Isn't it amazing God in His wisdom provided plants in the garden to aid us in cleaning our homes, and these plants serve to build and strengthen our immune systems while we clean?

These essential oils which serve to protect our health can be blended at home using therapeutic grade oils or purchased already formulated. Essential oils have been safely used for thousands of years; some of the oils are strong and must be diluted with carrier oil, such as olive oil, while others are gentle and can be used directly on the skin or swallowed.

I recall, as a child, my mom putting a few drops of clove oil in my mouth when I suffered with a toothache, and I remember how it gave me almost instant relief.

Let's all take a big step forward into the past and begin to use the essential oils from God's garden!

For myself, I have found essential oils to be useful in a multitude of ways. I prefer organic oils, unless I am using them for cleaning purposes, then I may choose a less expensive essential oil.

The recipe listed below is an age-old formula utilized for so many purposes, including cleaning purposes; used effectively long before manufacturers persuaded us to use their hormone disrupting products as cleaning agents.

Thieves' Oil Recipe

- 200 drops of clove oil (a powerful antioxidant)
- 175 drops of lemon oil (antibacterial and antiseptic)
- 100 drops of cinnamon bark (antifungal)
- 75 drops of eucalyptus oil (antibacterial)
- 50 drops of rosemary oil (analgesic and antiseptic)

This essential oil preparation should be stored in a dark glass container, away from heat and sunlight, preferably in a cool location.

Please note that one 15-milliliter bottle of essential oil contains approximately 250 drops, and one 5-milliliter bottle contains approximately 85 drops.

Household uses: The Thieves' oil can be used as an all-purpose spray for cleaning and disinfecting around the home, purifying the air, and eliminating odors, germs, bacteria and viruses—one drop of thieves' oil for each ounce of water. Add the oil first; then add water. It mixes better that way. Shake vigorously before each use or before spraying the mixture.

To clean cell phones, spray the mixture very lightly on a cloth, and gently wipe the phone. Spray pet beds. Spray mattresses to dispel bed bugs and discourage dust mites. Add six drops to laundry loads to help kill bacteria. Add six drops to dishwater to help kill bacteria. Add fifteen drops to a bucket of cleaning water. Use this wonderful combination of oils to clean countertops, furniture, steering wheels, and door handles as well as using it as a nontoxic hand sanitizer.

For topical application and massage: one drop of thieves' oil should be diluted in jojoba oil, or any carrier oil, such as olive oil or grape seed oil. Thieves' oil is too strong to apply directly to the skin. Massage into the feet, the lower back, the back of the upper legs, the neck, and behind the ears. This recipe is excellent for daily use as protection against germs, especially during the cold and flu season. This product helps to strengthen the immune system.

This essential oil should not be used directly on the skin of pregnant women, as it contains rosemary oil. The use of any oils on young children should be accompanied with caution and a generous amount of carrier oil in order to avoid burning tender skin. I learned that you should not administer essential oils orally to young children. Rosemary oil should be avoided by people suffering with high blood pressure.

I learned to use different variations of Thieves' Oil in a diffuser, an item I purchased from my local health food store. When I diffuse Thieves' Oil, it purifies the air in my home, eliminating cooking odors and other household odors. I also learned diffusing this essential oil formulation in my home can help combat a respiratory infection and help prevent a virus from spreading in my household.

I learned I could take Thieves' Oil internally, as well, and that it would help stop a cold in its tracks. I mix it with food or drink and take it multiple times a day. I have also heard a number of individuals claim this stopped the beginning of a cold.

Listed below are the ways that I have learned to use essential oils in my home. I have found I can safely use essential oils for my family and pets. Essential oils can be used three ways:

1. Aromatically: Inhale the oil's aroma either straight from the bottle or dispersed into the air, spritzed or diffused.
2. Topically: Apply directly on skin. Some oils may be applied neat (meaning with no dilution) while other oils need to be diluted with a vegetable oil before being applied to the skin.

3. Internally: Take an essential oil through the mouth. Oils may be placed in an empty capsule, taken with water or another form of liquid, or taken straight into the mouth. NOTE: Dr. Clark warned against administering essential oils orally to small children and pregnant women.

I learned that while most pure therapeutic-grade essential oils are gentle enough to apply to the skin when used properly, there are a few that can potentially cause discomfort (such as oregano or cassia). If an essential oil is strong and causes discomfort or heat when applied directly to the skin, it is important to always use a vegetable oil to dilute the essential oil. It is recommended that you just rub some vegetable oil right on the area of discomfort and to never use water to dilute the essential oil. Because water and oil do not mix well, water will not dilute it and can actually drive the essential oil deeper into the skin.

ESSENTIAL OILS

Frankincense: There is a saying among essential oils users: "When in doubt, use frankincense." This is because frankincense is good for everything! Frankincense is antibacterial, anticatarrhal (inflammation of the mucous membranes), anti-inflammatory, an expectorant, anti-carcinogenic, antitumor, antidepressant, anti-infectious, antiseptic, an immune stimulant, a sedative, cytophylactic (stimulating regeneration of the cells), a digestive, a diuretic, and an astringent. Frankincense has been studied all over the world for its anticancer properties. Nicole Stevens and others have published research on the anticancer effects of frankincense.

Frankincense contains sesquiterpenes that enable it to cross the blood-brain barrier (BBB) and help bring oxygen to cells in the brain. Frankincense may be used aromatically and topically for many things, including Alzheimer's disease, asthma, balance, brain injury, concussion, inflammation, liver cirrhosis, mental fatigue, and depression. It may be used topically for viruses of the nerves, warts, wrinkles, and moles. Frankincense may be used internally (via a capsule, in water, or directly in the mouth) as well as aromatically and topically for cancer. Warning to those in menopause—when I swallowed some drops of Frankincense during menopause, I experienced an instant hot flash.

Lemon: Lemon is awesome. It has been studied for its antidepressant effects. Just take a whiff, and you will know why. Lemon is uplifting, refreshing, and invigorating. Lemon essential oil contains compounds that dissolve petro chemicals. Add a few drops of lemon essential oil to your daily water intake to clean the petro buildup from your cells. (Be sure to use a glass or stainless steel container, rather than plastic, a petroleum by-product.) Apply directly to areas of cellulite to assist detoxification. Apply topically to treat cold sores.

Lemon can also help with constipation and sluggish digestion. Historically, lemon has been used for food poisoning, scurvy, lowering blood pressure, and liver problems. When using topically, avoid direct sunlight for up to twelve hours at the application site. Because of lemon essential oil's ability to aggressively dissolve petro chemicals, it is a wonderful degreaser and can be used to remove gum and other sticky or greasy substances. Add a few drops of lemon oil to some baking soda, and use it to clean the counters and bathtub.

Lavender: Lavender has many properties, including being analgesic, an antidepressant, an antihistamine, antifungal, anti-inflammatory, and a sedative. Lavender is fantastic for burns. When treating a burn, first place the burn in cool water to stop the *cooking*. Then apply several drops of lavender essential oil. Lavender is very healing to the skin and can be used for rashes and itching as well as treating fungus on the skin. Lavender is also very relaxing and is a calming oil to use before bed. Diffuse it, or apply it to the bottom of your feet to aid in relaxation. Place a cloth with a few drops of the oil on it inside of your pillowcase to inhale as you sleep. Lavender can be taken internally to help with allergies.

Melaleuca (also known as Tea Tree Oil): Melaleuca is a strong antiviral, antibacterial, antifungal, parasitic, immune stimulant, and more. Historically, the aborigines used leaves from the melaleuca tree to help heal cuts, scrapes, infected skin, and wounds. Melaleuca essential oil can be used topically for things like ear infections, staph infections, eczema, jock itch, and athlete's foot. Melaleuca can be diffused to combat airborne viruses and bacteria. Melaleuca may be taken internally to stimulate the immune system.

Peppermint: Peppermint is a favorite essential oil because it smells so great. But it is more than just a wonderful aroma! Peppermint oil is not only invigorating, but also antibacterial, anti-inflammatory, antispasmodic, and antiviral. Peppermint essential oil can aid with alertness; just breathe in the aroma and apply to reflex points. Inhale the aroma deeply to help with asthma and open the airways. Apply to cold sores to aid healing. Apply to the back of the neck and forehead for a cooling effect for fevers. Apply to temples and back of neck for a tension headache.

Applying peppermint to the temples and over sinus cavities will bring sinus headache and congestion relief. A drop of peppermint in water and a drop on the stomach can help with digestion. Dilute at a one-to-one ratio with vegetable oil when applying topically on sensitive skin or on children. Use peppermint with caution if pregnant and when dealing with high blood pressure.

Oregano: Oregano can be used to strengthen the immune and respiratory systems. It is antibacterial, antifungal, antiviral, and antiseptic to the respiratory system. It is also an immune stimulant. Dilute one drop of essential oil to three drops carrier oil (such as coconut oil) when applying topically. Dilute even more for young children. Oregano oil can be used topically for athlete's foot, carpal tunnel syndrome, parasites, ringworm, warts, whooping cough, MRSA, and for warming the body.

Oregano essential oil may be taken internally for intestinal germs, bacterium and fungal infections and as an immune system stimulant. To remove warts, carefully apply diluted oregano oil to the wart only (being careful not to apply to surrounding skin) several times a day until the wart falls off. Diffuse oregano essential oil when combatting viruses or bacterial infections.

A respiratory blend: My mom used Vick's Vapor Rub. Look for a blend containing bay laurel leaf, peppermint, eucalyptus radiate, melaleuca alternifolia, lemon, and ravensara. These oils fight against airborne bacteria and viruses. They are able to open up the respiratory system as well as soothe respiratory tissues. This blend can bring respiratory relief when nothing else seems to work. Rub a drop or two into the palms of your hands, cup them over your nose, and inhale deeply through the nose. Apply topically to the chest, back, and the bottoms of the feet. Inhale and diffuse at nighttime to breathe better for a more restful sleep. Dilute with vegetable oil (such as coconut oil) for sensitive or young skin.

A protective blend contains oils such as wild orange, clove bud, cinnamon bark, eucalyptus radiate, and rosemary. There is a claim that these oils help strengthen the immune system. Studies have proven there is faster healing in the mouth after dental work is performed when a protective blend is used. This blend can be used to kill bacteria, viruses, and mold. I use this essential oil blend in a diffuser or spray it into the air and also use it to disinfect and clean surfaces in my home. My dental hygienist mixes this blend with pumice to clean my teeth.

To make a spray, you will need a four-ounce glass bottle with a spray nozzle, vodka, a protective blend, and distilled water. Combine two tablespoons of vodka with twenty drops of protective blend essential oil in the bottle. Let them blend for ten minutes. Then top the rest of the bottle off with distilled water. Shake before each use. This combination can be sprayed into the air or used to clean surfaces.

To use a protective blend topically, I learned to dilute one drop of essential oil to fifteen drops of a carrier oil. While this blend may be applied to several areas of the body to stimulate the immune and lymphatic systems, it is best to apply it to the bottoms of the feet, because it may be caustic to the skin. Repeated use can cause extreme contact sensitization; avoid use during pregnancy. A protective blend can be mixed with carrier oil and taken internally in capsules to help with issues such as bladder infection, staph infection, and hypoglycemia.

A digestive blend will contain oils such as ginger, peppermint, tarragon, fennel, caraway, coriander, and anise. This particular combination of oils will soothe digestive system ailments as well as help balance the digestive system. Apply topically on the area of concern, and take internally to assist with the following: constipation, diarrhea, heartburn, upset stomach, nausea, parasites, colitis, and Crohn's disease. Apply one to two drops topically for bloating. This blend can be applied topically on the stomach. Do not use if you have epilepsy.

Essential oils can also help bring relief to muscle aches and pain. A blend of essential oils which sooth aches and pains will consist of oils such as wintergreen, camphor, peppermint, blue tansy, German chamomile, helichrysum, and osmanthus. These oils are anti-inflammatory, improve circulation, cleanse the blood, provide pain relief, and much more. A soothing blend helps address deep muscle and bone pain as well as problems with the nervous system. Apply topically for arthritis; fibromyalgia; joint pain; muscle aches, pains, or tension; inflammation; back pain; bursitis; and more. This blend can also be applied directly on the reflex points on the feet. A soothing blend should only be used topically. Repeated use may cause contact sensitization. Do not use on children and avoid use during pregnancy.

Cilantro Oil: This oil is often blended with other elements. Cilantro oil will remove heavy metals from the body. Metals in the body cause fungus to develop, creating a foundation for the growth of cancer.

I learned that in order for essential oils to be truly effective, they must be 100 percent pure, natural aromatic compounds that are skillfully derived from plant sources. I learned to choose essential oils that are totally pure and do not contain any fillers or artificial ingredients whatsoever. When essential oils are free of any contaminants, such as chemical residues or pesticides, their active therapeutic qualities are not diluted in any way.

THE IMPORTANCE OF A CLEAN ENVIRONMENT

Whoever first said cleanliness is next to godliness in benefiting humankind truly had a revelation. When God sent Jesus to redeem us from the curse of sin, somewhere along the line, the church took up the teachings of the New Testament and ignored the laws of the Old Testament, among them instructions on cleanliness. There is no denying this because a multitude of God-fearing men and women dispensed medical care for hundreds of years with complete disregard for the simple necessity of washing their hands before treating a patient.

Until relatively recently in history, the warning given in the Bible of the danger of fungi (i.e., mildew, mold, and yeast) was also ignored. There is now an increased awareness of the danger fungi pose to health and its link to the disease of cancer. As the result of living in our present information age, we can now take a look back through the Old Testament with a much greater appreciation of the wisdom God so graciously imparted to His people.

Careful attention to keeping the home environment and body clean comes with obvious benefits. Bacterium unchecked is capable of producing an enormous amount of disease and misery.

There are many simple steps we can take to ensure the growth of germs and bacteria in our environment is kept to a minimum. Aside from being diligent about keeping our hands washed and free of germs, keeping our hands away from our mouths helps to minimize the amount of germs which may enter the body and create sickness. We must be diligent about washing our hands before eating! One of the biggest ways disease is introduced into the body is by eating finger foods with unwashed hands and failing to wash our hands before putting our hands into our mouth.

Establishing the habit of removing the shoes upon entering the home is a habit which will actually have a positive impact on the health of the entire family, as this helps to eliminate exposure to outside toxins which were trodden through (i.e., herbicides, pesticides, and fossil fuels as well as bacteria, fungi, and germs). Carpeting holds a lot of toxins and though it may be an added expense, removing carpet from the home is a step in the right direction to achieving better health.

Sleeping on a fresh pillowcase each night—a simple measure to take—actually assists in keeping us healthy. Using a clean towel after each bath and not drying the face with the same towel used to dry the body helps to avoid germs and bacteria. Using clean kitchen towels at the beginning of each new day helps in avoiding germs and bacteria. Do not forget the powerful ability of the sun's rays to kill bacteria, as ultraviolet radiation is very effective in killing bacteria. Living in Florida means lots of sunshine; so I very frequently put bed pillows in the sunshine for the day.

Avoid placing an egg carton directly into the refrigerator, as it is a common source of bacteria; rather place eggs in a container and then refrigerate. It is extremely easy to contract illness from bacteria present on the outside of an eggshell. An egg carton is easily the dirtiest item at the grocery store; ask that your egg carton be bagged separately.

I have seen a couple of people develop a painful lump on the bottom of their feet. I learned from my friend Hannah the cause of this lump is bacteria contracted from eating a dirty egg. The remedy to treat this type of lump on the bottom of the foot is to use a colon cleanse. The lump will quickly dissipate!

North American Herb and Spice Company sells an excellent product called Oregamax, a blend of medicinal herbs. I learned that whenever a person is health challenged, Oregamax will protect from the potential side effects of eating eggs that are contaminated with bacteria. Oregamax is especially helpful to have on hand when eating in a restaurant. I have seen more than one very healthy person sickened as the result of eating eggs in a restaurant.

One of the most effective actions we can take to help keep our bodies cancer-free is to keep the mouth clean by flossing and brushing with a sterilized toothbrush. Either H202 or the Juice of Wild Oreganol can be used to sterilize a toothbrush, as can some essential oils. I learned that cancerous tumors begin in the colon, and the mouth is the doorway to our colon. The tumors then metastasize or spread to other areas of the body. Good oral hygiene is a key to protecting our health.

Finally, I also learned not to neglect changing the air filters in the home on a regular basis. A recommended guideline would be every 30 days. The air you are recirculating should be clean and toxin free; this is such an important part of good health. If you develop any sort of respiratory illness, i.e., a cold or the flu, change your home air filter immediately; you can actually recover from a cold much quicker.

CHAPTER 28

A Daily Must for Good Health

Enter you in at the narrow gate; for wide is the gate, and
broad is the way, that leads to destruction —Matthew 7:13

I learned through my experience a fundamental factor: If the diet does
not change—unless one begins to make healthy food choices—it will
not matter what supplements are taken; there will be no lasting recovery
from cancer. Maintaining good health requires a lifestyle change. I had
to begin eating nutritious food, allowing my body to heal, rather than
eating devitalized foods containing little or no nutrition, which are filled
with artificial ingredients hazardous to my good health. I learned eating
processed foods was akin to starving my body to death, preventing my body
from rebuilding, strengthening, or thriving. When I began to consume raw
vegetable drinks in my Nutribullet, I had so much energy!

On a daily basis, I take wild source vitamin C, such as rose hips, camu
camu, or pomegranate powder. I learned that eating pomegranate seeds
also provides a substantial amount of vitamin C. Wild source vitamin C
removes radioactivity and mold from the body. According to Dr. Clark,
our water supply is contaminated with radioactivity. This is damaging
to the cells, making us more vulnerable to cancer, and this results in
accelerating the aging process. Vitamin C will assist in preserving a
youthful appearance.

One tablespoon of sunflower seed butter or a handful of sunflower
seeds taken daily will provide a good source of selenium. Dr. Clark claimed
our kidneys are blocked or clogged with wheel bearing grease and motor

oil contained in city drinking water and manufactured food. Selenium unclogs or unblocks the kidneys by moving the wheel bearing grease and motor oils accumulated by the kidneys into the bladder, where they are then emptied out of the body through urination. This will help reduce hot flashes, as there is a connection between the kidneys being blocked by these substances and the hot flashes themselves, according to Dr. Clark. Dr. Clark tested many processed foods and found that they contained wheel bearing grease, motor oil, and isopropyl alcohol, which is used as a cleaning agent on manufacturing equipment—another reason to eat fresh! Selenium rounds up yeast in the body and delivers it to the kidneys. This is an extremely important fact to remember.

One or two Brazil nuts eaten daily will provide germanium to the body. Germanium removes chlorine from the body's cells. I learned that it is extremely important to do this on a daily basis, as Dr. Clark links the presence of chlorine in the body to the disease of cancer.

I now take one capsule of MSM daily, which breaks up any chlorine that I may have been exposed to throughout the day.

When a person has a persistent cough or a cold, I learned nuts should be avoided. If a person has a respiratory problem of any kind, I learned their daily germanium source should be two capsules of hydrangea root, and the daily selenium source should be three capsules of selenium, rather than eating seeds and nuts; all of these supplements can be purchased from www.ibeatcancers.com.

As the result of my research, I learned that vitamin C promotes the healing of wounds and aids in protecting the body against bacterial infection. I read that flushing the body with ascorbic acid will treat chemical allergies and chemical poisoning. I also learned that vitamin C will help rid the body of arsenic, which is often an ingredient of chemotherapy. Vitamin C is effective in treating radiation poisoning; antibiotic resistant bacteria; fungus; and the cancer I was waging war against.

I learned that if my health was really challenged and my budget allowed for it, I could see a physician who practices alternative medicine and request a prescription for a Myer's cocktail. The cocktail consists of vitamin C and essential vitamins B5, B6, B12, B complex, and calcium and magnesium. The B vitamins are essential to health as they resist yeast, a cancer-causing agent.

My sister took my mother for these treatments, and they gave her a tremendous boost in energy. Unfortunately, we were missing other keys that would have saved my mom's life.

I learned when one is very ill, constipation may be experienced. Rather than using harsh laxatives which deplete the body of nutrients, an ascorbic acid flush is recommended by Dr. James Balch in his book *Prescription for Nutritional Healing.* The ascorbic acid flush is one teaspoon of esterified ascorbic acid in an eight-ounce glass of water or juice taken every half hour. I learned I should keep track of how much has been taken until the stool is softened to a tapioca consistency. Although I learned this is a good remedy; I learned to be extremely careful, as too zealous an approach will lead to diarrhea. I found a slow and very patient approach will produce a much more agreeable result.

CHAPTER 29

A Lifestyle of Detoxification

Purge me with hyssop and I shall be clean. Wash me
and I shall be whiter than snow.—Psalm 51:7

I have mentioned a number of methods I employed to detoxify my body.
I learned that detoxification is the simple key to remaining healthy
throughout our lives. The body stores toxins it has absorbed through
the lungs, glands, skin, and digestive tract. Recognizing this and taking
measures to detoxify the body will help insure we can remain disease-free.
I learned neglecting to detoxify increases the risk of developing any disease,
not only cancer, as toxins weaken the body's immune system.

The body has its own ways of detoxifying—through exhalation,
perspiration, urination, and bowel elimination. However, the amount of
toxic chemicals in our environments have increased to such a degree that
the built-in methods of detoxification our Creator designed us with are
incapable of keeping pace with such a toxic overload.

I learned that routinely ridding the body of toxins removes the burden
on the body's immune system, thus allowing the immune system to
rebuild and remain in a strengthened condition; this also aids the body's
biochemical functions, enabling the digestive tract to work properly and
allowing cleansing deep within the body's core. I read that detoxification
helps relieve many diseases, including colitis, chronic fatigue syndrome,
multiple sclerosis, fibromyalgia, auto-immune diseases, and many other
modern-day maladies caused by a toxic overload.

I learned a premier method of detoxifying the body is far infrared sauna. It promotes a deep and healthy detoxifying sweat where toxins reside, at the cellular level. The body sweats out many toxic substances, including harmful germs, fungi, yeast and bacteria, as well as heavy metals. The far infrared sauna is useful in improving circulation, cleansing the skin, lowering blood pressure, aiding weight loss, and improving cardiovascular health. You will find a great selection of equipment, including far infrared saunas and the ion cleanse foot detox spa by going to www.ibeatcancers.com.

The ion cleanse foot detox spa is also an excellent detoxification tool, ridding the body of germs, bacteria, fungi, yeast and metals, as well as radiofrequency energy.

I learned that a colonic hydrotherapy session is a wonderful detoxification, as well. If your budget does not provide for these detox measures, then herbal cleanses are an ideal solution for you, along with daily exercise that produces a gentle sweat. I learned that even sunbathing can assist in detoxifying the body.

We all love the convenience of cell phones and other wireless devices, but the usefulness of these electronics does not come without a price, as they expose us to a form of electromagnetic radiation called radiofrequency (RF) energy. I learned that the body actually collects and holds this toxic positive energy. The effect this has on the body is the cells are destabilized, and cell mutation takes place, creating a vulnerability to tumor formation in the brain or other areas of the body where the radio frequency is penetrating. Researchers claim there is evidence that men who make a regular habit of keeping their cell phones in their pants pockets can have an increased risk of developing prostate cancer.

While reading an Internet article written on this topic, I happened upon a YouTube demonstration entitled "cell phone pops popcorn." What I viewed was a demonstration of individuals making a circle of three or four cell phones around kernels of popping corn, and when the cell phones began ringing simultaneously, the kernels began popping without any heat source whatsoever. This is a sobering situation. In one of the Internet articles I read, authored by a scientist who was warning of the seriousness of exposure to RF, he mentioned the danger of sleeping all night next to a cell phone.

It was my habit to store my cell phone in my bra when I went running—the exact spot where the breast tumor later developed. Obviously, this was not a very bright idea on my part.

There are methods available for us to combat the problem of the storage of RF energy in the body. Wild hibiscus tea contains a component that is helpful in cleansing cells, thus allowing the cells to be strengthened and stabilized.

In addition to the ion cleanse foot detox spa, which also removes toxic positive energy from the body, walking barefoot on the ground, a practice known as earthing or grounding enables the body to discharge the positive energy which has been collected. When bare feet touch the sand or ground, the earth transfers a supply of electrons to the body, which strengthens the immune system. The earth has a slightly negative charge; so as a person walks barefoot on the sand or the ground, electrons from the earth flow into the body, giving a virtual transfusion of healing power. Along with that is the added benefit of deeply breathing fresh air. Earthing or grounding reduces the positive charges our bodies collect from exposure to the electronics we are engulfed by in our modern society.

There is a documentary entitled, *The Grounded* and its sequel *The Grounded 2*. These two documentaries discuss how positive energy from electronics can easily rob our good health.

A Himalayan salt lamp aids to reduce the positive energy in the home caused by wireless electronics. The single most effective supplement which aids in counteracting the positive electrical energy collected by the body is wild source vitamin C. Purchase these products from www.ibeatcancers.com.

CHAPTER 30

Our Beautiful Feet

How beautiful on the mountains are the feet of
them that bring good news.—Isaiah 52:7

I learned that the condition of our feet is an indication of the state of our health. Problems in the feet are not to be ignored, as they are symptoms of deteriorating health. They are warning signals—flashing yellow lights—that indicate the kidneys are blocked, the immune system has been compromised by an overload of toxins, and heavy metals need to be removed in order to avoid more serious health issues.

Are the feet swollen? I learned that this should not be overlooked. Through my own experience, I learned the kidneys need to be detoxified immediately, as this type of swelling puts a dangerous strain on the heart, slowing blood flow. I read that along with kidney-cleansing herbs, and drinking lots of alkaline water, the detox trio of vitamin C, germanium and selenium, aids in unblocking and clearing the kidneys of accumulated motor oils and wheel bearing grease which have entered the body through such sources as treated drinking water and the ingestion of processed foods, as well as occupational exposure to oils and grease.

I learned that drinking adequate amounts of good, pure water and juicing organic vegetables for a few days while carefully avoiding sugars will also help to quickly flush the kidneys and remove swelling. Drinking herbal teas will aid the body in flushing toxins, according to Dr. Clark's book, *The Cure & Prevention of all Cancers*. Bell makes an excellent kidney cleansing tea.

I learned that as the result of gravity, the toxins the body accumulates over the years settle into the feet. This accumulation of metals, especially copper, leaves the feet prone to stubborn fungal infections in the toenails. I learned the Juice of Wild Oreganol will kill this fungus when taken three times a day for a month or longer; however, grains, fruit and all sugars must be avoided for it to be fully effective.

I learned that the herb pau d'arco taken daily also helps discourage the recurrence of fungal infection. I learned, however, it is necessary to adopt new eating habits to maintain health.

I learned that the first line of defense we have to protect our feet is footwear. The bottoms of our feet are portals or entryways to the entire body.

Our bare feet can pick up germs, bacteria and toxins in our environments. The shoes we wear should ideally have leather soles which actually aid in removing the positive electromagnetic energy which builds up in the body from the use of wireless electronics.

I also learned of homeopathic methods which may be employed to remove toxins from the body through the soles of the feet. The best method of this type of detox is the ion cleanse foot detox spa. This process involves pulling various toxins from the body, such as fungus, yeast or candida, heavy metals, germs, bacteria, acids in the joints and the harmful RF energy the body has collected from wireless electronic devices. I learned that this brings rapid relief to the liver, gall bladder, kidneys, lymphatic system, and joints. The ion cleanse foot detox spas are recommended for anyone suffering with painful joints, sciatica, migraines, hypertension, diabetes, acne, arthritis, depression, fatigue, as well as many diseases. Its ability to pull acids from the body can provide a significant reduction in joint pain.

This piece of equipment can be purchased through my website or an independently owned health food store should be able to give you information concerning a provider of this particular service in your area. Massage therapists and reflexologists often offer this foot detox as one of their services.

I learned that this is a tremendous detox for a person who is health challenged and well worth the expense. The cost is usually between

$25 and $60 per treatment, and many spas offer a reduced price when purchased in a package deal.

Because of the ion cleanse foot detox's ability to cleanse the bloodstream so quickly, a person will experience a renewed sense of energy and vitality after just one footbath.

Reflexology, as a medicinal practice, has been around for thousands of years and is used as a diagnostic tool in the practice of Eastern medicine. It is a type of massage based upon specific areas on the soles of the feet and palms of the hands which correspond to all of the lymphatic glands and the organs; including all regions of the body. Reflexology massage aids in opening the portals of the feet and hands, enabling the body to more efficiently release the toxins. It is best used in conjunction with the ion cleanse foot detox.

Reflexology is an excellent diagnostic tool for determining the state of one's health and in locating the particular organ which needs to be detoxified. A good reflexologist can easily pinpoint the exact area of illness in the body.

As the result of an automobile accident several years ago, I suffered with a herniated disc in my low back and was plagued with sciatica. I had chiropractic treatments and practiced yoga and Pilates and got a minimal amount of relief, but my symptoms eventually worsened and I began to experience pain and weakness in my foot if I drove my car for more than a half hour. After just one treatment of reflexology, followed by an ion cleanse foot detox, I experienced a significant reduction in pain, as the cleansing ions pulled pain-causing toxins from my body. I read some personal testimonies of others who had purchased the ion cleanse foot detox, and they also commented on being relieved of pain.

Another method used for detoxing through the feet is a Chinese homeopathic patch which can be purchased from a health food store or even sometimes a pharmacy. The patch is treated with wood vinegar essence made from medicinal trees and is applied to the soles of the feet, low back or any other part of the body where pain is experienced. The patch is worn overnight. While there is a removal of toxins with this method, it is not nearly as effective as the ion cleanse foot detox.

Kenkoh USA sells a massage sandal which helps to cleanse and detoxify based on reflexology. The sandals, which are meant to be worn for the first hour or two in the morning, have a thousand natural rubber nodules that gently massage the feet as you walk, dislodging accumulated uric acid crystals. The dislodged uric crystals enter the bloodstream and eventually pass out of the body in the urine. When worn consistently, Kenkoh sandals purportedly will help prevent gout. The nerve endings are stimulated, and the blood circulation is improved. The sandals aid in revitalizing the feet and rejuvenating the entire body as the result of detoxification. This is a great gift for the person who seems to have everything!

Besides aiding in improving the circulation, Kenkoh sandals are recommended for stress relief, neuropathy, edema, back pain, neuromas, bone spurs, sciatica, arthritis, tendonitis, heel pain, muscle soreness, tension headaches, numbness, metatarsal pain, swollen ankles, low energy, varicose veins, leg cramps, injury, sports recovery and, of course, gout.

I learned that all of these homeopathic methods will help relieve the body of contaminants and aid in restoring health. I read that it is important to remember to drink plenty of water and medicinal teas while employing any detoxification program. I mentioned before the importance of drinking enough water, but it bears repeating because of its necessity for the body's recovery. It is recommended that a person drink half of their body weight in ounces. For instance, if you weigh 120 pounds, you should drink 60 ounces of water daily, and the medicinal teas can also count as part of your fluid intake. Purchase the items I mentioned at www.ibeatcancers.com.

CHAPTER 31

To Eat or Not to Eat Meat

For the kingdom of God is not meat and
drink; but righteousness, and peace, and joy
in the Holy Ghost.—Romans 14:17

There is currently a trend of thought in our nation that has led many to adopt a vegan or vegetarian lifestyle, with the notion that their health will be increased and perhaps even that their lifespan will be lengthened. A true vegan eats mainly raw or dehydrated produce, seeds and nuts, while avoiding meats, dairy products, and eggs; while a vegetarian avoids meats but continues to eat eggs and dairy products.

At Hannah's suggestion, I initially ate a vegan diet. She told me that eating a strict vegan diet would help to rapidly cleanse my lymphatic system.

Since that time though, I have had the opportunity to read many books on alternative medicine and even sit under the teachings of some very bright people in this nation—leaders on the cutting edge of the alternative medicine movement, and they have all said the very same thing: Eating a strict vegan diet long term will eventually break down the body.

I learned from these people that eating organic, grass-fed beef and other free-range meats, as well as wild meats, will actually strengthen and protect the body from developing cancer. I learned that these meats will aid in speedily healing a body stricken with cancer or any other disease.

I learned that when eating meat, I must make sure to supplement the meal with enzymes, which reduces the burden on the digestive tract and pancreas and strengthens the body.

The most important thing Dr. Clark stressed about eating meat is it must first be cooked until it falls off the bone—whether it is wild meat, beef, lamb, chicken, turkey or fish—in order to avoid germs and bacteria. I learned that broth which has been made by slowly cooking the bones is very nutritious and will help speed recovery from an illness. I learned that I should avoid eating raw fish while battling cancer. This is extremely important. Uncooked or undercooked meat or fish can quickly reintroduce germs and bacteria into the intestinal tract, according to Dr. Clark.

I learned that if I ate meat during the healing process, that it would be important for me to make sure I had regular bowel movements, not to allow myself to become constipated. I learned constipation causes a buildup of bacteria and fungi in the intestinal tract.

I learned to avoid eating barbequed or grilled meats! A quick search on the Internet reveals the link between eating barbequed or grilled meats and the disease of cancer. I learned eating meats cooked in this fashion can very quickly break down the immune system.

When the dietary law was given to Moses in the Book of Leviticus, God gave instructions on which animals were considered as clean and could be consumed and which animals were considered unclean and were to be avoided. God would not have permitted eating meat in the dietary law if eating meat was in any way bad for your health. However, I learned it was vitally important that the meats I did eat needed to be raised in a healthy environment. Pork and shellfish are among the meats which God classified as unclean and were to be avoided, which meant God knew something about these meats that was bad for our health.

I have a young friend in her early twenties who shared with me she was plagued by recurring urinary tract infections; almost as soon as one cleared up, another one surfaced. She was constantly taking antibiotics. I told her this was linked to what she was eating, and we discussed her diet. I mentioned she should avoid eating pork products, as they are linked to chronic urinary tract infections. She told me she ate bacon on a daily basis but would stop.

Several months later, since eliminating bacon from her diet, she had not had a single urinary tract infection.

I learned that the meat I do eat should not be cooked in any sort of non-stick pot, but rather stainless steel, glass, enamel or a crockpot. I learned I could also use a cast iron skillet, but that I should avoid using a microwave.

During the healing process, I learned it is a good idea to wear disposable plastic gloves when handling raw meat in order to avoid contamination, as one can contract germs and bacteria from handling raw meats, especially when the immune system is challenged.

I learned to avoid eating lunch meats or hotdogs during the healing process, as these meats have been found to be heavily laden with harmful estrogens, germs and bacteria, as well as cancer-causing chemicals. As a health conscious person, I now avoid eating this type of meat products.

I also learned that I should completely avoid farm-raised fish, as it contains high concentrations of PCBs and dyes—cancer-causing agents. I learned that the introduction of PCBs into the body will cause the health of a sick person to deteriorate very rapidly. Within five to ten minutes of eating this kind of fish, I can tell I have eaten something toxic. I learned to not mistakenly think it will not hurt if I eat it just once. I now make sure any fish I eat is wild caught or farm-raised in a fashion that is not toxic to me! I learned I could eat canned wild caught salmon, tongol tuna (purchase this online at www.ibeatcancers.com) and sardines.

Additionally, I learned to completely avoid shellfish. Shellfish filter the toxins in seawater; therefore, they are a toxic food source and should not be eaten even occasionally, according to Dr. Clark. A weakened immune system is unable to tolerate these toxins. Just one shellfish meal could mean a severe setback in health for a person whose immune system is already weakened. Shellfish are associated with leaky gut, a condition that will invite germs to enter the bloodstream.

CHAPTER 32

Recipes

O taste and see that the Lord is good: blessed is
the man that trusts in him.—Psalm 34:8

After addressing the disease of cancer with the herbal germ cleanse and carefully avoiding exposure to isopropyl alcohol and chlorine, as well as not eating plants in the allium family, I learned the single most important thing I could do to improve my health is to begin cooking. I learned to cook fresh food.

Now, if I want to eat dessert, I make it myself using almond or coconut flour.

If I want to eat ice cream now, I use an ice cream freezer, using organic cream, raw cacao powder, stevia and vanilla to make it myself. If I want salad dressing, I make it from healthy ingredients. You get the picture. The healthiest meals are the ones prepared at home.

I learned to focus on preparing meals which include lots of vegetables! I started cooking!

If you feel bewildered by the task, search the Internet. You will be healthier and live longer when you begin to eat foods made from fresh ingredients.

I certainly did not set out to write a cookbook, but I felt it was important to include some recipes which would be of help in getting you started—recipes I wish I would have had when I faced cancer. For the best results during the healing process, I learned to eat a lot of vegetables, lightly steamed and eat salad greens, such as romaine, spinach, baby kale, and arugula, giving them a punch with grated ginger, tomatoes and sesame oil; and I started adding nuts and seeds to my salads for some crunchy satisfaction. I drank lots of raw vegetables that I whipped up in my Nutribullet. I love raw kale; it gives me so much energy.

It is so important to remember that not all vegetables should be eaten raw. I learned that cruciferous vegetables, such as Brussels sprouts, broccoli, cauliflower and cabbage are great cancer fighters, as they reduce the amount of dangerous estrogens. Rather than raw, though, I learned that cruciferous vegetables should be eaten lightly steamed.

The exception to this rule is eating fermented cabbage, such as sauerkraut, kimchi or cabbage rejuvelac. I also learned that all squash should absolutely never be eaten raw, but always fully cooked or dehydrated.

I learned that while pursuing good health and detoxifying the body, I should eat very simply.

For breakfast, I began with my homemade rejuvelac and then ate my special granola. I have included both recipes for you. For lunch and dinner, I ate sugar-free sunflower seed butter with a sprinkle of Himalayan pink salt on celery, adding some hemp seeds, also called hemp hearts, which have amazing anti-cancer properties. I sprinkled them liberally on the sunflower seed butter.

The following nutrient-rich traditional fats have nourished healthy population groups for thousands of years: Butter; beef and lamb tallow; lard; chicken, goose, and duck fat; coconut and palm oils; cold pressed olive oil; fish oils. Dr. Clark recommended these fats and just recently I have read on the Internet that these foods are healthy after all.

In many of my recipes, I use Himalayan pink salt; this salt contains important trace minerals. Celtic sea salt is another good salt for the body, as it contains both sodium and potassium, which jointly share the task of reducing high blood pressure.

I learned that it is the opinion of many who practice alternative medicine that all salt is not bad for the body. However, sodium hydrochloride, marketed as table salt, is absolutely toxic to the body and should be avoided. This harmful salt is poisonous to the body and breaks down the immune system. Sodium hydrochloride is also found in processed foods. This is just one of the reasons processed foods must be avoided in order to successfully rebuild health. The secret to recovering our health is rebuilding the immune system.

If you do not have a dehydrator to make the flaxseed cracker recipe, do not despair, as I have included a delicious flaxseed bread recipe which can be baked. This bread is delicious! My husband even likes this bread, so I can boast the Rock household seal of approval. Most importantly, eating this bread will get the flaxseed moving in your colon and pushing out all of the toxins. Make absolutely sure you stay hydrated with plenty of medicinal teas or water when eating this flax bread.

Even though I chose not to eat dairy during the healing process, I have included the method of sterilization of dairy products. I learned that a person who is extremely ill with the disease of cancer may need the dense calories organic dairy provides in order to regain their strength, but I learned the dairy must first be sterilized in order to prevent the reintroduction of dangerous germs into the system. Later on, I learned that adding a few drops of 35% H202 to a glass of milk will be equally effective in sterilizing the milk.

Sterilization of Milk

Boil one pint of milk with a pinch of salt for ten seconds. Allow the milk to cool to room temperature. Add 1/8 teaspoon of powdered vitamin C and 1/8 teaspoon of aluminum-free baking soda, and stir. This may be consumed immediately or refrigerated for later use.

Dairy products should be at least 2 percent fat to enable calcium absorption. A person who is ill should definitely consume sugar-free, whole fat dairy products.

Sterilization of Butter

Bring one pound of butter to a boil in a saucepan with a pinch of salt. Boil for ten seconds, and add just a pinch of vitamin C. Add an equal amount of olive oil. Reheat, and pour into a bowl. Discard any liquid that accumulates at the bottom. Refrigerate until ready to eat.

Cabbage Rejuvelac

Start by putting the chopped cabbage and distilled water in the blender. Start the blender at low speed and then advance the blender to high speed. Blend for 10 seconds or less. Do not over blend.

Pour the blended mixture into a squeaky clean quart jar that has a tightly fitting lid. Allow 1 inch of space at the top of the jar, which makes room for expansion.

Keep the jar at room temperature, below 72 degrees Fahrenheit. After 3 days, 72 hours, strain the liquid rejuvelac and place the liquid into a clean jar. The cabbage may be discarded.

Use ¼ cup of the fresh rejuvelac liquid to make your second batch of rejuvelac, which takes only 24 hours. Place chopped cabbage and 1½ cups of distilled water into the blender. Begin at low speed and advance to high speed, blending for 10 seconds. Again, be careful not to over blend.

Pour the mixture into a clean quart jar, adding the ¼ cup of rejuvelac you previously made, leaving at least 1 inch of space for expansion. Screw the cover on tight, shake and let it stand 24 hours. Strain the mixture, reserving ¼ cup for new mixture. Immediately refrigerate excess rejuvelac for drinking.

Discard any rejuvelac on hand after 24 hours. Avoid using tap water because the chlorine will interfere with the production of the bacteria. Either boil the tap water for 30 minutes or let the tap water sit in an open container for 24 hours before using it to make rejuvelac.

Good quality rejuvelac tastes similar to a cross between carbonated water and the liquid whey obtained when making yogurt. Bad quality rejuvelac has a much more putrid odor and taste. Do not consume foul smelling rejuvelac!

Drink ½ cup of cabbage rejuvelac 3 times a day, preferably with meals.

SOUP

Homemade soup can be a safe and nutrient-packed meal for a person who is ill. Make sure that you use no processed ingredients—e.g., bouillon cubes, soup starters, or commercially made chicken broth, as it is packaged in aluminum. Salt is to be added during the boiling process of the meat, not at the end. This raises the boiling temperature and kills bacteria, according to Dr. Clark. Adding vinegar (just a dash) draws the calcium out of the soup bones, supplying an extra boost of nutrition.

Anti-Cancer Chicken Soup

Cooking time for the chicken is about 3 hours and allow 1 hour for vegetables to cook.

- One large stainless steel soup pot
- One organic or free range chicken
- Enough water or organic chicken broth to cover the chicken
- 1 tablespoon of white or apple cider vinegar
- 2 or 3 teaspoons of Pink Himalayan Salt
- 2 or 3 stalks of celery
- 4 large tomatoes
- 1 eggplant
- 3 carrots, peeled and chopped
- 1 small bunch of rapini or kale chopped and precooked
- ¼ of a purple cabbage, sliced as thin as spaghetti noodles
- 2 turnips chopped into bite-sized pieces
- 1 large thinly sliced zucchini or 2 small ones

Place chicken in pot and cover with liquid, adding salt and vinegar. Bring to a boil and then reduce to a simmer. Simmer chicken until well done; chicken parts are easily pulled apart. Remove the chicken from the broth and place in a bowl to allow it to cool.

Add to the broth chopped celery and chopped tomatoes. Peel the eggplant and chop into bite size pieces and add to the pot. Bring to a slow boil and cook for 15 minutes or until the vegetables are softened. Then add carrots, turnips and purple cabbage and continue to cook 15 minutes longer on medium heat.

Add zucchini slices and cook on medium heat until zucchini are thoroughly cooked, about 10 to 15 minutes. Add precooked rapini and heat until warm.

Separate chicken from skin and bones and chop into bite-sized pieces, add to soup and stir.

Dr. Clark's Cheesy Chicken Soup

- 4 cups homemade chicken broth
- ½ cup minced cooked chicken
- ¾ pound uncolored cheddar cheese, cut up, purchase from the health food store
- ¼ teaspoon vitamin C
- 1 teaspoon freshly grated nutmeg or other spice of your choice
- 2 cups of cooked butternut squash chunks
- Cooked celery, chopped (optional)
- 1½ cups cream or half and half (no need to boil)
- Himalayan pink salt

Make sure the butternut squash and celery have been pre-cooked by boiling. Bring all ingredients to a boil. After one minute, turn the heat to low, cover the pan, and simmer for at least 20 minutes, stirring frequently to prevent the soup from sticking to the bottom of the pot.

Creamy Butternut Squash

- 1 butternut squash
- ¼ cup unsweetened almond milk or milk
- Ground coriander
- Ginger
- 1 egg, well beaten

Preheat the oven to 350 degrees.

Cut a large butternut squash in half, and scoop out the seeds in each half. Place the two halves on a baking sheet, placing the cut side of the squash up, and bake for approximately one hour, until very soft and tender when pierced with a fork. Let the squash cool, and carefully peel the skin away from the squash flesh. If placed in the refrigerator to completely cool, the squash is much easier to peel.

After you have peeled away the outside skin and discarded the stem, place the squash flesh into a food processor along with ¼ cup of unsweetened almond milk, and pulse repeatedly until creamy. You may add less or more unsweetened almond milk, depending on the size of the squash, being careful not to make it too runny. Add coriander and ginger to taste. This recipe helps satisfy the desire to have something creamy, smooth, and sweet.

Baked Butternut Squash

This savory recipe is my favorite but the most work to prepare. It is delicious and will help keep you satisfied.

- 1 large butternut squash
- Olive oil
- Himalayan pink salt to taste
- Preheat oven to 350 degrees.

Peel a large butternut squash. This is not the easiest of tasks, but I have found that I can best achieve peeling the squash by first cutting each end of the squash off, then cutting the squash in half where the neck and the large part of the squash meet, and then holding it upright make downward strokes with a potato peeler. After peeling it, cut the squash in half and scoop out the seeds. You can save the seeds in the refrigerator for another recipe.

Dice the peeled and seeded squash into bite-sized pieces or long strips like French fries, and place on a very lightly oiled baking sheet.

Drizzle olive oil over the squash, sprinkle lightly with salt and toss so it is evenly coated. Bake until tender.

Toasted Squash Seeds

- Raw seeds from a butternut squash or pumpkin
- Himalayan pink salt
- Olive oil or grape seed oil

Preheat the oven to 400 degrees. Clean all squash debris from the seeds, and place seeds on a baking sheet. Sprinkle the seeds with salt and then drizzle a very small amount of oil over the seeds. Mix the seeds by hand until they are well coated with the mixture.

Bake until the seeds are brown. Watch them closely so as not to burn them. These seeds are very satisfying and crunchy as a snack, tasting pretty close to popcorn.

Crunchy Granola

- 1 small handful raw walnuts, chopped
- 1 small handful raw almonds, chopped
- 1 small handful raw sunflower seeds
- 1 small handful hemp hearts
- 1 small handful shredded raw coconut

Place all ingredients into a bowl, and toss together. Store in a glass dish, covered in the refrigerator. Serve in a cereal bowl with added almond milk. This is a good breakfast and can also be packed for an on-the-go snack.

Almond Flour Pancakes

- 1/3 cup of almond flour
- 1 egg
- A pinch of Himalayan pink salt
- Almond milk or milk
- Coconut oil

Beat the egg and pinch of salt together, adding the almond flour and just a splash of milk or almond milk. Stir the batter until the consistency is that of regular pancake batter, not too thick, adding more milk if necessary. Heat a cast iron skillet on medium heat, adding a teaspoonful of coconut oil to the hot pan. When the skillet is hot spoon small amounts of the batter onto the pan, making small pancakes. When small bubbles appear at the top of the pancakes, carefully flip the pancakes and cook a couple of minutes longer. Serve with poached eggs and butter.

Rosemary Flaxseed Crackers

- 2 cups of golden flaxseeds
- 3 cups of purified water

- 2 cups of raw almonds
- 1 teaspoon of Himalayan pink salt
- ¼ cup fresh rosemary, coarsely chopped

This recipe requires a dehydrator. Finely grind the flaxseeds in a coffee grinder. Soak the ground flaxseeds in the purified water for one hour. It will become gelatinous. Grind the almonds in a food processor, then add the ground flaxseeds, salt and finely chopped rosemary into the food processor until it is well blended.

Spread the cracker mixture on dehydrator trays lined with parchment paper as evenly as possible, without leaving any holes and not spreading it too thin. Dehydrate the crackers at 115 degrees F for approximately 6 to 8 hours. Flip the cracker mixture and dehydrate for another 3 to 4 hours. Break the sheet of crackers into smaller pieces and continue to dehydrate for another 6 to 10 hours.

Sometimes I make this recipe using cumin and chili powder, rather than rosemary. It's a satisfying and crunchy cracker.

Flaxseed Bread

This awesome bread is baked focaccia style because it is baked flat on a sheet pan and then cut up into whatever size pieces you choose. It is a palatable way to get flaxseed in the diet. It works great for toast, sandwiches, and other bread uses (e.g., pizza). It is rough in texture, like heavy whole grain breads, but the carbohydrate in flax is almost all fiber. Drink lots of water with this bread, and avoid eating too much all at once. Its high fiber content can easily lead to gas and bloating. It would be advisable to eat small portions of this bread with digestive enzymes!

- 2 cups flax seed meal
- 1 tablespoon aluminum-free baking powder
- 1 teaspoon salt
- 5 beaten eggs
- ½ cup water
- 1/3 cup of olive oil or coconut oil

Preheat the oven to 350 degrees. Use parchment paper that has been lightly oiled on both sides to line two baking pans.

Mix the dry ingredients well with a whisk. Beat the eggs very well by hand in a separate bowl, add the water and oil, and mix again. Combine the wet and dry ingredients, making sure there are no strings of egg white. Let the mixture set for 2 to 3 minutes to thicken. Do not leave it longer than 3 minutes, or it will become too difficult to spread.

Pour the batter onto the two pans equally. Because it's going to mound in the middle, spread the mixture away from the center, and you will get a more even thickness. Spread into a rectangular shape, staying an inch or two away from the sides of the pan.

Bake for about 20 minutes until the bread springs back when you touch the top and/or it is visibly browned. Cool and cut into whatever size slices you choose. This bread can easily be cut with a spatula.

Place the bread on a cookie sheet and add a light sprinkle of oregano, add a few spoonsful of pizza sauce, and sprinkle generously with your choice of cheese; heat in a warm oven at 350 degrees for just a few minutes, and you now have a tasty pizza.

Add a light dusting of ground coriander and powdered stevia on top of a slice of this bread, and you've got yourself something that tastes very similar to a donut!

My favorite way to eat this is topped with a poached egg and a side of cooked spinach.

Savory Raw Beet Salad

This delicious salad will help satisfy a craving you may have for meat. My husband, who is a big man with a hearty appetite, loves this salad and considers it a full meal. I ate this salad nearly every day during my healing process, never tired of it, and still love it. Eating raw beets helps to cleanse the liver.

- 2 raw beets, peeled
- Small slice of ginger, finely grated or chopped
- ½ ripe avocado
- 2 cups arugula greens

- Olive oil as dressing
- Himalayan pink salt to taste

Optional Additions

- 1 handful raw sunflower seeds
- 1 handful raw walnuts
- 1 handful raw pumpkin seeds
- Raw hemp hearts
- 1 tablespoon ground flax seed

Shred the beets in a food processor. Place the shredded beets into two individual serving bowls, and top with ginger, chopped avocado, walnuts, pumpkin seeds, and ground flax seed. Dress with a drizzle of olive oil and a sprinkle of pink salt and sunflower seeds and/or hemp hearts.

Raw Tacos

- Several leaves of romaine lettuce washed and dried
- ½ cup of chopped tomato
- ½ cup of chopped ripe avocado
- ¼ cup of shredded carrot
- 1 cup of raw walnuts, chopped
- Cumin
- Himalayan pink salt
- (Optional) Add well-cooked, grass-fed ground beef

Mix the tomatoes, avocados, carrot and walnuts and sprinkle with cumin, adding salt to taste. Fill the romaine leaves with the mixture and eat like a traditional taco.

Avocado Boats

- 1 ripe avocado
- ½ cup raw walnuts, coarsely chopped

- ½ cup of shredded raw beets

- Olive oil
- Himalayan pink salt

Cut the avocado in half lengthwise, and gently give it a twist to separate the two halves. Remove the seed by striking with the sharp edge of a knife. Once the knife is anchored in the seed, turn the knife sideways, and the seed will pop out. Lightly salt the avocado, and then fill with walnuts and beet mixture. Dress with olive oil, and enjoy.

Mexican Skillet

- 2 chopped zucchinis
- 1 chopped tomato
- 1 package of chopped shitake mushrooms
- 1/4 grated carrot
- 1 handful of walnuts
- Chili powder
- Himalayan pink salt
- Olive oil or coconut oil
- (Optional) Add well-cooked, grass-fed ground beef

Add a small amount of oil to a medium hot skillet and fill with zucchini and tomato. Sauté until the vegetables are softened, adding mushrooms halfway through the cooking process.

Sprinkle in cumin and salt to taste. Stir in chopped walnuts and plate immediately. Garnish with avocado and grated carrot.

I also add eggplant to this dish and use oregano and basil, rather than cumin. This makes for a delicious Italian skillet.

Kale Chips

- 1 bunch kale, torn into one-inch pieces (Wash the kale well and dry in a salad spinner or dry with paper towels for best results.)
- 3 tablespoons olive oil
- 1 tablespoon of apple cider vinegar
- ½ teaspoon Himalayan pink salt

Preheat the oven to 400 degrees.

Whisk the oil and vinegar, and toss the kale in the dressing until coated but not overly saturated.

Place kale pieces on a baking sheet that has been covered with parchment paper, and very, very lightly sprinkle with Himalayan pink salt.

Bake for 10 to 15 minutes until crispy. You can turn the kale over halfway through the baking process for crispier results.

These chips taste exactly like the yummiest commercial potato chips, but they are so much better for you!

Green French Fries

- 1 pound green beans
- Olive oil
- Himalayan pink salt

Preheat oven to 400 degrees.

Wash and clean the green beans, and dry thoroughly. I use a salad spinner for this process. Place the green beans on a baking sheet. Sparingly add salt and a drizzle of oil. Mix together by hand, and spread evenly on the baking sheet, trying to give each bean its own space. Bake 10 to 15 minutes until lightly browned, remove from oven, and turn the green beans over with a spatula. Return the green beans to the oven until lightly browned.

The next few recipes are desserts that should be reserved until your health has improved. They are great options for those who want to avoid sugar, but still crave sweets. The sweetener in these recipes is stevia. When you are cooking with stevia, less is better. Adding too much stevia to a recipe will produce a bitter, distasteful dish.

Stevia Sweetened "Peanut" Butter Cups

- 1 cup of raw pecan halves
- 1 cup of unprocessed shredded coconut
- ½ teaspoon of Himalayan pink salt
- ½ cup of culinary coconut oil
- ½ teaspoon of liquid stevia

- ¼ teaspoon of vanilla extract
- 3/8 of a cup of unsweetened organic sunflower seed butter
- 3 teaspoons of Psyllium husk
- 1 package of paper baking cups, like you would use to make cupcakes

Mix the pecans, coconut and salt in a food processor until well blended. Scrape the sides and add the remaining ingredients. Mix in the food processor until well blended. Pour a small amount of the mixture into a baking cup, about a ½ inch and freeze.

Chocolate coating:

- ½ cup of culinary coconut oil
- 2 ½ teaspoons of raw cacao powder
- ¼ teaspoon of vanilla extract
- 4 drops of liquid stevia

Mix the coconut oil with the stevia in a small dish and then blend in the cacao powder. Frost each frozen "peanut" butter cup quickly with the chocolate topping, as it will harden very fast. Store in the refrigerator; makes about a dozen cups, depending on the desired thickness.

This recipe can very easily be switched up to make different flavors of candy. Omit the sunflower seed butter and instead add several drops of peppermint oil, an essential oil. Add a few drops at a time and taste before adding any more of the peppermint oil, as it can easily become overpowering. I love the combination of orange and chocolate. To make this flavor, omit the sunflower seed butter and add orange oil, also an essential oil, in place of peppermint oil. Omit the sunflower seed butter and cacao coating and add lemon oil, an essential oil, for lemon squares.

PIE CRUST OR COOKIE RECIPE

This versatile recipe can be mixed with raw cacao chips for a "chocolate chip cookie" recipe or used with different essential oils to achieve different flavors

This recipe will also make a great crust for a berry pie or a delicious apple Betty recipe.

Basic recipe:

- 1 and ½ cups of almond flour (the best kind of almond flour has had the skins on the almonds removed before grinding)
- 5 tablespoons of organic extra virgin coconut oil
- ¼ teaspoon of vanilla
- Several drops of stevia (remember that less is more)
- Optional: add unprocessed shredded coconut

Mix all of the ingredients in a food processor until it sticky dough is created. If making a fruit pie, press the dough ball evenly into a large pie dish. Heat oven to 350 degrees and bake in a hot oven for 15 to 20 minutes, depending how thin you have made the crust, watching it closely to make sure it doesn't burn. After the pan has cooled, place it into the refrigerator.

- 3 cups of berries
- ¼ cup of water
- A few drops of stevia
- ¼ teaspoon of vanilla
- 1 teaspoon of agar agar

Place the berries of your choice into a saucepan with a small amount of water on medium heat. After the fruit has softened, add stevia and vanilla. Reduce the heat to low and remove a small amount of the juice and mix with agar agar. Stir until agar agar is dissolved and return the mixture to the saucepan for a few more minutes. Pour mixture onto pie crust and store in refrigerator until cool. For best results, this pie should be kept cold before serving.

For apple Betty, follow the same recipe and add apples and cinnamon. Reserve some of the dough for the top of the apple Betty. Pour the apple mixture over the baked crust and place small bits of the dough directly onto the apple mixture. Return to oven and remove when the top is brown.

If choosing to use the recipe to make cookies, pinch off a small amount of dough and roll into a ball, flatten the ball onto a cookie sheet and bake in an oven that has been preheated at 350 degrees. Bake for about 10 minutes and store in the refrigerator.

CHAPTER 33

The Importance of Washing Raw Produce

Wherefore come out from among them, and
be ye separate, says the Lord and touch not
the unclean thing.—2 Corinthians 6:17

I have come to understand that eating raw produce in salads and drinking raw vegetable smoothies or juicing raw vegetables—such as carrots, beets, and greens—will feed the cells, speed healing, and help to provide boundless energy. Although preparation, particularly when juicing, is time consuming and requires a lot of cleanup, my efforts are rewarded in a multitude of healthy ways. Raw carrot and beet juices aid in swiftly rebuilding my immune system and assist in ridding my body of dangerous cancer-causing germs. I found that juicing greens eliminates constipation and delivers the nutritional needs of the body.

In her books on healing cancer, Dr. Clark warned that carrots should not be consumed by those with liver cancer.

I did not juice at all while battling cancer, but I did drink vegetable smoothies I whipped up in a Nutribullet and my recovery was speedy. If you do choose to juice or make vegetable smoothies, there are some things which are important to remember, such as eliminating germs and protecting your health.

This is what I learned: All non-organic produce should first be ozonated for 7 minutes in a bucket of water before consumption. According to

Dr. Clark, this process safely removes the xeno estrogens, the harmful pesticides sprayed on non-organic produce in order to kill insects. I learned that xeno estrogens are particularly dangerous for someone suffering with a hormonal cancer. Following this step, Dr. Clark suggested adding one drop of food-grade iodine (Lugol's iodine) per one quart of water in the bucket. The produce should be submerged in the solution for at least one minute in order to destroy germs. There is no need to ozonate organic produce, but even organic produce should be treated with the iodine solution before eating it raw. I learned it was very important to AVOID juicing non-organic produce if a person is suffering with cancer, particularly a hormonal cancer.

I learned it is important to rinse the produce thoroughly before preparing. According to Dr. Clark, neglecting this step can re-introduce cancer-causing germs into the body very quickly during the healing process. Once the immune system has been compromised and cancer established, vigilance is key. It is a small price to pay for the opportunity to live many more years with strength and vitality. The future is in the hands of the diligent. When the immune system is properly strengthened, the body should then be able to fight off disease.

Dr. Clark also warned that vegetables must be carefully cleaned when prepared for raw juice consumption. Carrots and beets should be peeled and washed thoroughly. Carrots are prone to the infestation of carrot weevils, which typically bore into the tops and sides of carrots, requiring close inspection for the weevils' telltale holes. Otherwise, the carrot juice may contain the weevils and their eggs. Failing to thoroughly peel and clean root vegetables that are consumed raw can introduce deadly pathogens into the body. Because root vegetables are washed and peeled, it is not necessary to submerge them in iodine. I remember eating small red radishes and becoming very ill. I learned through this experience that I should avoid eating anything that grows beneath the ground but is too small to peel. I read that eating bitter vegetables, such as a radish, is extremely beneficial, so I now eat the larger Daikon radishes which are easy to peel.

I learned that it is best to avoid dining out while battling cancer. However, if it cannot be helped, I then would avoid eating any raw foods when dining out. I have come to understand that cooking simple home-cooked meals, using healthy ingredients, is the best way to get well.

So many restaurants today microwave pre-packaged food that contains high amounts of salt and many unhealthy additives. One of the books I read while doing research stated you are far less likely to develop cancer in the first place when you avoid dining out.

If you miss dining out, consider taking turns hosting dinners with friends or hire someone who's a great cook or even a caterer to come in and prepare a meal for you on the weekends. Whenever I start feeling like cooking is drudgery, I watch the cooking channel for inspiration and then make healthy versions of the recipes I've seen.

CHAPTER 34

Treating Pets with an Herbal Germ Cleanse

*As the deer pants after the water brook, so my
heart yearns for you, O God—Psalm 42:1*

As much as we love our pets, they can be a major source of germs, viruses and bacteria entering our home. I am vigilant about having my 8 pound Maltese, Zsa Zsa Pinks, groomed and bathed. When I pick her up from the groomer, she always has two pink bows on her head, and her fluffy white coat looks beautiful. However, when I take her outside she needs to be on a leash, as she delights in rolling in the dirt or, even worse, sniffing the feces left by another animal. She isn't at all discriminating. As dearly as I love her and as much effort as I take in keeping her clean, she still remains a source of germs, viruses and bacteria. Because of what our pets may encounter on a daily basis outdoors, it is extremely important to always make it a practice of washing our hands after handling pets!

As the result of our pets tracking germs, viruses and bacteria into our homes, the likelihood of our developing cancer actually increases, and even more so when we have several pets in the household. When someone is ill with cancer, Dr. Clark stated it is vitally important to also treat their pets with the herbal germ cleanse. In her book, Dr. Clark shared stories of successfully treating pets for cancer.

The User Guide with the recommended dosages for treating pets can be found at www.ibeatcancers.com. As a pet lover myself, I know this may call for some effort, but Dr. Clark states in her book, *The Cure & Prevention of all Cancers,* it is a matter of life and death for the cancer sufferer to eliminate germs, viruses and bacteria from the home environment.

Dr. Clark recommended asking someone to board your pet in their home for 3 weeks and administer the herbal germ cleanse initially. She stressed that when your pet returns to your home 3 weeks later, you must continue administering a small amount of the herbs on a daily basis.

Dr. Clark's recommended dosages for treating pets with an herbal germ cleanse is available on my website, www.ibeatcancers.com.

I didn't ask someone to keep my little dog when I was ill, but I did give her Dr. Clark's suggested herbal germ cleanse. I am also vigilant about washing my hands after handling her.

Dr. Clark urges that you not sleep with your pet, and to not even sleep in the same room as a pet when you are ill with cancer. I understand this can be a difficult undertaking, as I have a difficult time telling my affectionate little dog no when she wants to snuggle up in bed with me during a thunder storm. She wins every time.

However, if you choose to follow Dr. Clark's sage advice, I have discovered the best solution to this problem is the use of eucalyptus oil lightly diffused in the bedroom. Both dogs and cats find the smell of eucalyptus oil to be offensive, and using it is far better than having to continually scold a beloved pet. When eucalyptus is present my dog chooses to sleep in another room.

A pet should be bathed at least once a week, according to Dr. Clark, and most especially when we are health-challenged, in order to control the presence of germs, viruses and bacteria. Miracle II Soap with moisturizer is an excellent product for pet bathing, as it serves to kill harmful germs, viruses and bacteria, without harming you or your pet.

SECTION 5

Product Information

CHAPTER 35

Relieving the Side Effects of Chemo & RadiationTherapy

I will restore health to you and heal all
of your wounds– Jeremiah 30:17

I did not have any conventional medical treatment for cancer, and my health was fully restored using only the natural products listed in this book. Yet, recognizing there are individuals who may have already chosen the path of conventional medicine and may be considering boosting or supplementing their treatment, I am including suggestions offered by a physician to aid them in their journey. There are products available which offer protective support of the body while pursuing good health.

According to Dr. Cass Ingram, founder of the North American Herb & Spice Company, these are products which have proven to be effective in lessening or eliminating the damaging and permanent side effects of traditional cancer treatments.

Cranflush is one of these recommended products produced by the North American Herb & Spice Company. It is made from wild cranberries, includes other proprietary ingredients, and reportedly aids in preventing damage to healthy tissue during chemotherapy treatments. If I made the choice of chemotherapy, I would have several bottles on hand, and I would take Cranflush before, during, and after the treatment.

Additionally, I would take the Juice of Wild Oreganol, another North American Herb & Spice product. According to Dr. Ingram, this product has also been found to greatly aid in protecting the cells during chemotherapy treatments, as well as fending off the disease.

I would take the Juice of Wild Oreganol 3 times a day, mixing 3 tablespoons in low sodium V-8 Juice. I learned that wild oregano reduces the level of iron in the body, which is highly beneficial as excessive iron levels cause cell damage as we age.

I would also supplement with capsules of the spice turmeric also known as Curcumin, along with a lymphatic cleanse product, 3 or 4 times a day during conventional cancer treatment, as I learned this will boost the effects of conventional cancer treatment.

If I made the decision to have radiation therapy, I would use a product called Intestinal Drawing Formula made by HealthForce Nutritionals. This product contains kelp and zeolite and will aid in drawing radioactive material to the colon, allowing it to be expelled through the bowel, which greatly aids in helping to minimize any further toxicity to the body. After taking this product, I would have colonic hydrotherapy.

Chaga is a medicinal mushroom which is commonly used in Europe to curb the side effects of radiation therapy. Chaga Black, a product of North American Herb & Spice, is a wonderfully pure chaga mushroom drink with wild source vitamin C.

North American Herb & Spice also makes chaga creams which can be applied directly onto the skin. I also learned about Nutra Ultra Relief Cream, an MSM based cream, which is extremely useful in relieving and quickly healing the painful burns associated with radiation therapy.

Dr. Ingram reports that with the exception of the North American Herb & Spice product Chaga, which should not be used while being administered antibiotics or chemotherapy, all of the supplements and products listed in this book can be safely used during chemotherapy or radiation therapy.

These are effective whole food products, not medications with a long list of deadly side effects. All of the above-mentioned products can be located at www.ibeatcancers.com.

CHAPTER 36

Products I Used to Beat Cancer

I shall not die, but live, and declare the works
of the Lord.—Psalm 118:17 KJV

Initially, like almost everything else in life, this seemed a bit complicated, but soon all the pieces came together for me. I pressed on and achieved amazing results very quickly! I could tell a difference the very first day!

The dosages needed for the first 8 items were the most important, and I explained how I used them in Chapter 19, "An Eighteen-Day Herbal Germ Cleanse."

1. Wild source rose hip vitamin C
2. Hydrangea root
3. Selenium
4. Green black walnut capsules and tincture
5. Wormwood or Super W
6. Cloves
7. Ornithine
8. Ground flax seed
9. Castor oil— I used this as an oil pack over the tumor; I learned it softened the outer membrane of the tumor so the other products could more easily penetrate and dismantle the tumor; aids in rebuilding the immune system.
10. Arginine— one in the morning for energy and again at lunch
11. Hand sanitizer, must be isopropyl alcohol-free

12. Betaine hydrochloride— one with each meal; aids in digestion; Dr. Clark said betaine hydrochloride will stop diarrhea due to bacteria. Betaine hydrochloride also aids in ridding the body of candida.

13. Turmeric— two capsules three or four times a day with the lymph cleanse.

14. Lymph cleanse— two capsules three or four times a day; I used a product from Solaray.

15. A combination of calcium, magnesium and vitamin D. (Vitamin D rebuilds the immune system.)

16. Apricot kernels—see the chapter on "The Mighty Apricot Seed."

17. Miracle II Soap, Miracle II Neutralizer, and Miracle II Neutralizer Gel

18. pH strips to monitor pH levels

19. Clear Lungs by Ridgecrest Pharmaceutical— I took two or three every few hours when I developed congestion in my chest that I could not otherwise shake.

20. Vira Stop and Digest Gold from Enzymedica Therapy— I took one each with every meal

21. Beta Glucan—by NSC Immunition, I took as directed on the bottle; this marvelous product helps protect and rebuild a weakened immune system.

22. Lugol's iodine

23. Food-grade hydrogen peroxide – I later learned how to use this product on a daily basis to maintain good health. I explained this in Chapter 22.

24. Juice of Wild Oreganol

CHAPTER 37

The Mighty Apricot Seed

And God said, Behold, I have given you every herb bearing seed, which is upon the face of all the earth, and every tree, in the which is the fruit of a tree yielding seed; to you it shall be for meat.—Genesis 1:29

Amygdalin, a substance found in the seeds of fruit, nuts and edible seeds in varying amounts, is powerful and highly effective in the fight against cancer. According to Dr. Clark, the seed found inside of an apricot kernel contains the highest level of amygdalin, making it an excellent weapon in the hand of anyone battling cancer.

Dr. Clark wrote in her book, *The Cure & Prevention of all Cancers*, that the six fresh apricot seeds a day method can be used in conjunction with the herbal germ cleanse to reduce the recovery time from the disease of cancer. The use of these seeds will aid in very quickly removing any alkylating oils which allow the cancer-causing germ to flourish in the body. The apricot seeds literally help to starve the disease of cancer out of the body.

You can purchase the seeds and other products made from the apricot kernels, such as skin creams and Amygdalin B17 capsules from www. ibeatcancers.com. Amygdalin aids the liver in processing and eliminating toxins from the body. The skin creams are potent and can easily burn tender skin. I was unable to tolerate the Amygdalin B17 capsules, as they made me nauseated, but I know of others who tolerated them very well.

I have experienced excellent results with the apricot seeds, but I kept the number I ate to a limit of 6 seeds as Dr. Clark suggested.

I learned from Dr. Clark that apricot seeds should not be stored in the freezer, but that they may be stored in a cool dry place or refrigerated for up to a year before they lose their effectiveness. She recommended that you use nutcrackers to remove the seeds from the kernels, and that you begin by eating no more than 6 seeds a day. Apricot seeds contain a small amount of cyanide, but the level of cyanide is not enough to cause you bodily harm, according to Dr. Clark.

One alternative health care physician wrote that it is perfectly safe to eat 10 a day and that eating 40 a day is therapeutic, meaning that dosage amount could be used alone as a cancer cure therapy. I would not take this many seeds unless I was under the care of a physician who was familiar with apricot seeds. It is extremely important to gradually increase the number of the apricot seeds eaten, and it is recommended the apricot seeds be eaten by spreading them throughout the day, rather than all at once. When I ate more than 6 seeds, I experienced a very mild sense of lightheadedness, nothing severe, but I realized that the seeds were causing the light headedness. When I stopped eating the seeds, the lightheadedness disappeared.

If dizziness, headache or nausea is experienced, it is recommended that you decrease the number of seeds you are eating.

The following are the instructions Dr. Clark gave with regard to apricot seeds as a curative for cancer:

After cracking open six apricot kernels and removing the seeds, place three of the seeds in a coffee grinder. You can also grind these seeds by using a hammer; hammering the seeds while they are enclosed in a couple of plastic baggies. If very sick, Dr. Clark recommends that you choose the larger seeds—at least the size of the thumbnail. Grind the seeds, adding a dash of freeze-dried barley powder or some organic coconut flakes to make the grinding easier. Grind the ingredients for three seconds, stir them around, and grind for another three seconds. Put the mixture in a small bowl, and blend with a small amount of organic coconut oil or unsalted organic butter. Form into a suppository, and place into the freezer on a dish. Make this a daily ritual rather than making several suppositories at once.

Right before bedtime, when the suppository is completely frozen, grind an additional three or more seeds, again mixing it with just a dash of organic coconut flakes or freeze-dried barley powder before grinding, if desired. Immediately eat the prepared mixture, and then using a latex glove lubricated with Miracle II Gel insert the frozen suppository deep into the rectum.

Be sure to time the entire process so that the seeds are eaten and the suppository is inserted at approximately the same time; then retire for the evening.

Dr. Clark recommended that you repeat this process for two more days, and then take a break. Take one or two days off and repeat until feeling better.

If the 6 seed method is used in conjunction with the herbal cleanse, your body will detoxify very quickly. For this reason, Dr. Clark says it is extremely important to take extra precautions to protect from detox illness by being diligent about taking the detox trio, as well as enemas or colonics and drinking plenty of medicinal teas. I have provided a list of medicinal teas Dr. Clark recommended in Chapter 41 entitled "Medicinal Herbal Teas: Keys to Long Life."

I found the seeds which had already been removed from the kernel by the manufacturer were not as potent. If I was planning to dine out and could not be one hundred percent sure I was dining on foods free of alkylating oils, i.e., garlic, onion and the like, I found I could include these seeds in a smoothie or just eat them plain; they aren't too terribly bad, tasting a bit like almonds.

According to Dr. Clark, this is a simple, completely effective and inexpensive method which can be used on a daily basis to prevent the body from developing the disease of cancer again.

Later on, I learned taking 35% food grade hydrogen peroxide would accomplish the very same results.

CHAPTER 38

The Amazing Miracle II Products

Say to them that are of a fearful heart, be strong,
fear not: behold your God will come with a
vengeance, even God with a recompense; He
will come and save you.—Isaiah 35:4

Following my amazing recovery from cancer, I was introduced to some remarkable products produced by the Miracle II Company. Miracle II Neutralizer, an inexpensive bioenergy product, is beneficial to the body due to its ability to help quickly reach a healthy level of alkalinity in the bloodstream, allowing the body to heal itself.

The soap produced by this company is non comedogenic, meaning it does not clog the pores of the skin. Miracle II Soap and Neutralizer, as well as a number of other stellar products they produce, are pure and I learned are remarkably effective in ridding the body of harmful germs, viruses and bacteria which may remain in the body after the herbal germ cleanse. Remember, when the body is unburdened, it will naturally heal.

If I had an open wound from a tumor, I would use Miracle II Soap and Neutralizer mixed with distilled water to wash the wound. I would rely on the Miracle II products for bathing, as they are completely effective in eliminating germs, viruses and bacteria. Contrariwise, I learned that washing an open wound with any product containing isopropyl alcohol will increase the severity of the disease.

In order to restore and maintain good health, the Miracle II Company recommends you begin by drinking seven drops of Neutralizer, plus 2 to 3 drops of Miracle II Soap, in water every morning and evening, gradually increasing the amount of Neutralizer.

According to the company, these dosages of Miracle II products help effectively combat yeast infections, provided there is a strict adherence to an antifungal diet, a diet which is void of sugar, fruit or grain and also that Miracle II Soap and the Miracle II Neutralizer will help prevent a yeast build-up in the body.

Drinking several drops of Neutralizer on a daily basis helps to maintain the body's alkalinity at a healthy level. I learned that when using any product that increases the body's alkalinity, it is important to use pH test strips to monitor the alkaline level of the body. These test strips are available at better health food stores or a pharmacy. I read the recommended pH level of your morning saliva should be 7.36 to 7.44 to support optimum health. I read that the test should be performed the first thing in the morning, before eating or drinking.

I learned I could check my pH by dipping the test strip in my saliva collected in a plastic spoon. When the pH level dips below these levels, the bloodstream is acidic and accommodating to a multitude of degenerative diseases, including cancer, osteoporosis, osteoarthritis, kidney stones and heart disease. When the body is acidic, the liver produces more cholesterol.

When you are fighting disease, it is of utmost importance to maintain a proper alkalinity in the bloodstream.

The reason it is necessary to closely monitor your tested pH level is to avoid raising the alkaline level of your bloodstream above 7.44. It is detrimental to your health to become too alkaline. There is actually an illness, alkalosis, which causes heart palpitations and muscle twitching, among other symptoms, such as nausea and diarrhea, when the alkaline level in the bloodstream becomes too high.

Miracle II Neutralizer is an awesome product and when properly taken, I found it improved my overall health. I read about a young boy who was unable to have a bowel movement. His mother took him to see a physician who practices alternative medicine. After examining the child, the doctor recommended that he drink a few drops of Miracle II Soap and

2 ounces of Neutralizer in a glass of water. The child passed a dead tape worm the next day.

I have read accounts of individuals who healed themselves of cancer using Miracle II Neutralizer. This product has no offensive taste and would be ideal to give to children and the very ill. There are accounts of people who drank water mixed with Neutralizer throughout the day, in addition to following an antifungal diet, and after a few weeks, were able to leave a hospice facility and return home. This product is appropriately named, as taking it can produce miraculous results.

The Neutralizer quickly helps take the body's pH to a healthy alkaline state. Cancer, as well as other degenerative diseases, requires an acidic system to thrive. I learned that when the body is in a proper state of alkalinity, a tumor will no longer grow. Instead, the tumor begins to weaken and dissipate. Miracle II Soap, Moisturizer Soap and Neutralizer kill the cancer-causing germ!

All of the Miracle II products are useful in a multitude of ways and promote good health. The gentleman who created these products stated the formula was given to him during a night vision from the Lord. I listened to his extraordinary testimony on Youtube.

The Miracle II products would be an excellent addition for anyone interested in creating a "disaster relief or emergency survival pack," preparing for the possibility of any kind of disaster, such as storms, earthquakes, et cetera. I would definitely include the Juice of Wild Oreganol and the Oil of Oreganol in the disaster relief pack, as well. If someone was suffering with a bacterial infection and medical care was unavailable, these products could definitely prove to be lifesaving.

I studied the User Guide with great interest when I first purchased the Miracle II products. Not long afterward, I had a weekend guest in my home who mentioned she was suffering with a vaginal bacterial infection. She had waded up to her waist through polluted water rescuing a beloved pet during a tropical storm a few days earlier. She knew it was bacterial, rather than a yeast infection, as she had learned from an Internet search a bacterial infection will emit a fishy odor.

She planned to see a physician after the weekend so she could get started on an antibiotic, which was the solution recommended in her Internet search.

247

When she shared her predicament with me, asking if I could recommend a local doctor, I immediately thought of the Miracle II products. I recalled reading in the User Guide, which came with the purchase of my Miracle II products, the Miracle II Neutralizer was recommended for use in issues with bacteria. I suggested she give it a try, hoping it would give her a bit of relief until she saw a physician. She was more than willing to give it a shot because of the accompanying vaginal itching, which had left her in a miserable state.

She soaked, as directed in the User Guide, in a hot bath with the recommended amount of Miracle II Soap and Neutralizer, drank two ounces of the Neutralizer in a glass of water, along with 3 drops of Miracle II Soap, and douched with two ounces of Neutralizer mixed with four ounces of distilled water. Because she got immediate relief, she stopped using the products, and the symptoms returned in a few days.

She resumed the use of the products as before, but for a longer period of time, taking hot baths and douching two times a day for a full five days, as well as drinking the Neutralizer and a few drops of Miracle II Soap twice daily as before, just to make sure there were no lingering bacteria. She was healed completely without any necessity of antibiotic treatment!

This was positive proof for me these wonderful products are powerful and effective in ridding the body of harmful bacteria. I remember reading that the harmful bacterium produced by the disease of cancer is what brings death. For this reason I realized that ridding the body of dangerous bacteria is essential.

Miracle II recommends beginning by drinking very small doses of the Neutralizer—several drops to begin with, when using it as a prophylactic, meaning a measure to protect good health. However, my houseguest had no unpleasant side effects when she took the larger dosage recommended by the User Guide as a remedy for bacterial infection.

As the result of firsthand experience with the effectiveness of these awesome products, I quickly grasped how valuable they would be in the fight against cancer, even in advanced cases! As I said previously, if I had an open wound as a result of cancer, I would wash the wound with these products in order heal the wound and to avoid developing any further infection. If there was an infection, the products would be very efficient in eliminating it. I would bathe with the products, as well as drink them mixed with distilled water in order to heal the wound.

I read that when one can avoid antibiotics to treat a bacterial infection, the immune system is not further compromised. It is essential to remember that without a healthy immune system, there will be no recovery from disease.

These outstanding Miracle II products have a multitude of uses. In addition to ridding the body of toxins and their usefulness in personal hygiene, the products are recommended for defending plants against disease and a multitude of other uses. They are healing to the body and, according to company, can even be used to heal bedsores and help quickly rid the body of yeast infection! Drinking water with Neutralizer on a daily basis helped eliminate my hot flashes!

This company makes Miracle II Soap and Moisturizer Soap, a great body soap and shampoo; liquid Neutralizer; Neutralizer Gel, which can be safely used as a body lubricant and beauty treatment for the face, as well as toothpaste. They also produce a wonderful lotion; and a laundry ball that affects the electrical potential of the water, cleaning clothing with energy rather than chemicals, with added vinegar and baking soda serving to whiten the laundry, eliminating the need for chlorine bleach as a whitener.

Miracle II recommends applying a small amount of Miracle II Neutralizer Gel under the arms and then applying a non-aluminum deodorant stone over the gel. I found this to be a very effective and safe deodorant. Miracle II sells a deodorant stone, as well as a pump spray deodorant.

Purchase all of these products at www.ibeatcancers.com. These products truly are heaven sent!

CHAPTER 39

The Importance of Enzymes

He delivers the poor in his affliction, and opens their ears in oppression.—Job 36:15

I learned that enzymes are found in all living cells. They are biologically active proteins necessary for all living organisms. Metabolic enzymes are catalysts that regulate every biochemical reaction occurring within the human body, making them essential to cellular function and overall health. Digestive enzymes break down the food we eat, turning it into energy and maximizing this potential energy for use in the body. Translation: no enzymes, no energy!

I learned the pancreas releases digestive enzymes as they are needed by the body for proper digestion. The food we eat contains enzymes and mixes with our saliva, which also contains enzymes and then sits in the upper stomach approximately 30 to 45 minutes, where it is predigested and empties into the lower stomach. When the food reaches the lower stomach, a healthy pancreas excretes enzymes which help the food to further digest. When we eat overcooked, irradiated and processed foods, the enzymes have been destroyed, and therefore food is not properly predigested as it enters the lower stomach. This results in digestive discomfort.

I learned that a long term practice of these poor eating habits results in a breakdown in our health. The pancreas is overworked, as it must produce extra enzymes to aid digestion, and this drains enzymes from the pancreas, accelerating the aging process. After years and even decades of the pancreas being burdened by this process, the pancreas becomes weakened and its ability to excrete enzymes is greatly decreased. It is at this point that the body is unable to fight cancerous cells by utilizing its own storage of enzymes.

Secondly, I learned that this poorly digested food irritates the gut, and as a result food particles then leak into the bloodstream. This happens most particularly when there is leaky gut as the result of fungal overgrowth, brought about by eating too much sugar, particularly high fructose corn syrup, as well as other refined carbohydrates. This partially digested food which has leaked into the bloodstream is now treated as a toxin by the immune system. When this takes place, there is a sudden increase in white blood cells in the gut, as the immune system works to eliminate this toxin. This places a strain on the immune system, ultimately leaving the body weakened and vulnerable to cancer and other diseases.

Thousands of offending germs challenge our immune systems on a daily basis. Enzymes protect the body from these invading germs. When the levels of enzymes are high, the offending invaders are kept in check, and there is no disease.

However, when there is a deficiency in enzymes due to a lifestyle of poor eating habits, disease then becomes the dominant force. For this reason, supplementing with enzymes is essential in order to recover from illness. There have been reports of individuals being healed of cancer merely by the consistent use of proteolytic enzymes, along with eating a healthy diet.

Those who practice alternative methods to heal cancer will tell you the quickest and most effective method of achieving a healing from cancer is to eat a diet of steamed vegetables or dehydrated raw vegetables. When meat is eaten, the body utilizes its enzymes to break down and digest the meat. However, when limited amounts of meat are eaten or meat is avoided altogether, the enzymes instead break down and digest a tumor that is present in the body.

I learned that avoiding grains is necessary during the healing process, as grain contains an enzyme inhibitor, which prevents the enzymes from effectively dismantling a tumor.

While searching the Internet and reading various books and publications, trying to find out just what it took to break down a tumor, I learned that taking proteolytic enzymes on an empty stomach assists in dismantling the hard protein exterior of the tumor, as well as the tumor itself. I read that after taking proteolytic enzymes on an empty stomach, it is best to wait at least a full hour before a meal because when food is in the stomach, the enzymes instead break down the food rather than the tumor.

Proteolytic enzymes break down proteins; lipase breaks down fats; and amylase breaks down carbohydrates. I learned that taking a variety of enzymes is important.

The Enzymedica Company has a fine reputation as a producer of quality products. Its product Virastop contains a high content of protease, the powerful proteolytic enzyme. I took Virastop when battling cancer.

I had the opportunity to watch a television interview with the president of the Enzymedica Company. He mentioned he had a website that offered health advice on an individual basis at no charge. He said God had blessed his company, and he saw this as an opportunity to bless others.

Dr. Clark recommends taking digestive enzymes with meals to aid the digestive process. Digest Gold and Repair Gold by Enzymedica are outstanding digestive enzymes.

I found the product Wobenzym to also be an excellent source of enzymes. I found taking regular doses of enzymes on an empty stomach not only helped dismantle the tumor, but also provided relief from inflammation and pain in the body. I learned it was important to take enzymes consistently, but not in high doses. Rather, small doses should be taken frequently. For example, a small amount of enzymes an hour before a meal and a small amount of enzymes with a meal.

Because of the Wobenzym product's ability to heal scar tissue, they are also recommended for women who may be suffering with infertility as the result of scar tissue. The recommended therapeutic dosage of Wobenzym to rid scar tissue is 6 to 8 tablets on an empty stomach, first thing in the morning, with an ounce of sugar-free noni juice. I use Genesis noni juice.

Wobenzym is an enzyme derived from beef, and I learned it is a great product for those with blood type O. I learned that all other blood types should use plant-based enzymes.

Another excellent enzyme product I used was Bromelain, an enzyme derived from the core of a pineapple. I found Bromelain to be very effective if I had any sort of indigestion problem. These products are available on my website, www.ibeatcancers.com.

The foods that contain the highest amount of enzymes are figs, papayas, and pineapples. The center core of a pineapple contains the largest concentration of enzymes in the fruit. Since Dr. Clark recommended that you refrain from eating fruit when suffering with cancer, I learned it is best to rely on enzyme supplements. Enzyme supplementation is a key to slowing the aging process and remaining healthy.

CHAPTER 40

The Juice of Wild Oreganol & Oil of Oreganol

Ask and it shall be given you; seek and you shall find; knock, and it shall be opened unto you.—Matthew 7:7

I must list the many recommended uses of the Juice of Wild Oreganol, the awesome product I learned about which quickly extinguished the breast and rectal cancer threatening to take my life. The wild oregano bush, which grows among the rocks in the countryside of Greece, is simply a bouquet of love bestowed on all of humankind by the creator God. This powerful product obliterates many types of viruses, and destroys all germs, bacteria and fungi; it also has high antioxidant powers, making it a curative which strengthens the body's immune system, rather than breaking it down.

Dr. Cass Ingram established the North American Herb & Spice Company after being cured of the AIDS virus using oregano oil. His first experience with oregano oil was when a woman he worked with, who recognizing that he was dying, researched natural cures and hastily had a vat of the oil shipped to his door.

The Juice of Wild Oreganol is the most potent herbal germ-killing complex known which offers full safety to the body. It obliterates the influenza A virus and the human coronavirus.

According to Dr. Ingram, wild oregano has a positive effect on blood sugar and will help guard the body against the development of diabetes.

It eradicates MRSA as well as destroying noxious chemicals and is a key antidote to any toxin, including manmade chemicals, making it an excellent tonic to take during chemotherapy treatments and a remedy for recovery from the harmful side effects of chemotherapy.

Long term use of wild oregano may affect the body's ability to absorb iron, but this may be one of the reasons it is so effective in fighting cancer, as I learned an iron supplement should not be taken by a person suffering with cancer. Excessive iron in the body causes cell damage as we age.

When my husband suffered a stroke and was placed on life support, his hands and feet swelled. I massaged his swollen hands and feet with oregano oil and the swelling completely subsided in the space of only a few minutes. It is an amazing substance. My husband made a miraculous and full recovery, but that is another book!

The following is a list of diseases the Juice of Wild Oreganol is useful in treating. Whenever the recommendation is to apply topically, the reference is to Oil of Oreganol, and it can be diluted with carrier oil, such as olive oil, before applying it to the skin, particularly when applied to tender skin. The North American Herb & Spice Company markets oregano oil as Oil of Oreganol and Oil of Oreganol Super Strength. I prefer the Super Strength.

Oil of Oreganol may be taken internally as well. The Oil of Oreganol is sold in gel caps or may be placed in empty gel capsules. When I suffered a serious cut to my hand, I took capsules of Oil of Oreganol for 5 days to avoid developing an infection. I later learned that treating with 35% H202, as outlined in Chapter 22, would also serve to provide positive results when it comes to many of the diseases listed below because of its ability to cleanse germs from the body.

- Alopecia: drink the juice.
- Allergies: drink the juice
- Alzheimer's/Parkinson's disease: drink the juice.
- Amoebic dysentery: drink the juice.
- Ankylosing spondylitis: apply the oil topically and drink the juice.
- Antidote to any internal poison/venomous bite: apply the oil topically and drink the juice. (See a physician immediately.)
- Arthritis: apply topically and drink the juice.
- Autism or ADD: drink the juice.

- Bladder infections: drink the juice.
- Boils and goiters: apply the oil topically and drink the juice.
- Breast cancer: drink the juice.
- Broken bones: to speed healing, apply the oil topically and drink the juice; the hothouse featured in Chapter 45 will speed the healing of cuts and broken bones.
- Bromhidrosis (fetid body odor): drink the juice.
- Bronchitis: drink the juice.
- Bruises and injuries: drink the juice and apply the oil topically.
- Burns, including sunburns: apply the oil topically and drink the juice.
- Candida: take oil capsules, 2 capsules 3 times a day
- Canker and cold sores: drink the juice.
- Cellulitis: apply the oil topically and drink the juice.
- Chronic fatigue syndrome: drink the juice.
- Cirrhosis: drink the juice.
- Clostridium bacteria: drink the juice.
- Colds and flu: drink the juice.
- Colitis or irritable bowel: drink the juice.
- Congestive heart failure: drink the juice.
- Corona virus: drink the juice.
- Cryptosporidium and giardiasis: drink the juice.
- Dandruff: apply the oil topically.
- Diverticulitis: drink the juice.
- Ebola: take very high doses of Oreganol oil capsules and drink the juice
- Endocarditis: drink the juice.
- Epstein-Barr virus, cytomegalovirus: drink the juice.
- Fibromyalgia: drink the juice and apply the oil topically.
- Fire ant bite, spider bites, and bee stings: apply the oil topically.
- Food poisoning: drink the juice
- Gangrene: drink the juice and apply the oil topically.
- Genital herpes: drink the juice.
- Hashimoto's disease: drink the juice.
- Hepatitis: drink the juice.
- Indolent ulcer: drink the juice.

- Jaundice (quickly reversed): drink the juice.
- Kidney failure: drink the juice.
- Kidney infections: drink the juice.
- Kidney stones: drink the juice.
- Leg cramps/pain: drink the juice.
- Leukemia or lymphoma: drink the juice.
- Leukoplakia: drink the juice.
- Lou Gehrig's disease (ALS) and multiple sclerosis: drink the juice.
- Lumbar disc disease: drink the juice.
- Lupus/scleroderma: drink the juice.
- Lyme disease: drink the juice and follow the entire method of beating cancer in this book.
- Lymphedema: drink the juice.
- Lymphoma: drink the juice
- MRSA: drink the juice
- Muscular atrophy: drink the juice.
- Osteoporosis: drink the juice.
- Polycystic ovarian disease: drink the juice; avoid wearing gold metal on the body.
- Pneumonia: drink the juice, along with Clear Lung Extra Strength
- Psoriasis and eczema: apply topically and drink the juice.
- Pyorrhea (gum disease): drink the juice.
- Purification: drink the juice.
- Rosacea: apply the oil topically and drink the juice.
- SARS and the human corona virus in vitro: drink the juice.
- Scabies: apply the oil topically and drink the juice.
- Seborrhea: apply the oil topically and drink the juice.
- Shingles: apply the oil topically and drink the juice.
- Sinusitis: apply the oil topically to the outside of the nose and drink the juice.
- Sjogren's syndrome: drink the juice.
- Skin parasitic infection: apply the oil topically and drink the juice.
- Skin cancer: drink the juice, in conjunction with resveratrol and apply hemp oil topically to the affected area.
- Splinters: apply the oil topically.
- Stomach and duodenal ulcers: drink the juice.

- Thrush or vaginitis: drink the juice or take the oil in capsules.
- Thyroid cancer: drink the juice.
- Tick bite or attached tick: apply the oil topically and drink juice.
- Toenail fungus or athlete's foot: apply the oil topically and drink the juice.
- Toothache: drink the juice; apply clove oil for pain.
- Vaccination reaction: apply the oil topically and drink the juice.
- Varicose veins: drink the juice along with wild source Vitamin C and resveratrol.
- Vitiligo: drink the juice.

CHAPTER 41

Vitamin Supplements

*Where your treasure is there will your
heart be also. —Matthew 6:21*

I found that a daily regimen of these supplements supports my immune
system.

Supplement	Description/Type	Amount Per Day
Calcium	Calcium citrate or Calcium Made from Eggshells	If I eat dairy products, I take 300 mg calcium once a day. If I do not have dairy, I take 300 mg twice a day.
Magnesium	Magnesium citrate	If I eat dairy, I take 350 mg once a day. If I have not eaten dairy, I take 350 mg twice a day.
Cod Liver Oil	Cod liver oil liquid or capsules for Omega 3 (EPA plus DHA) & vitamins A and D; cod liver oil will aid in rebuilding the immune system	My dose varied according to the brand – the goal is to take a dose that provides these nutrient levels: Vitamin A: 20,000 – 30,000 IU Vitamin D: 800 – 1,200 IU Omega 3 (EPA plus DHA): 2,000 – 3,000 mg

Vitamin B Complex OR Nutritional Yeast "Flakes" *See more about Niacin below.	Balanced 50 mg tablets or capsules, plus Niacin (B3) if the product contains niacinamide (synthetic form), or Nutritional Yeast "Flakes," i.e. Red Star, Frontier, KAL, Now Foods Brand	I took 50 mg twice a day, plus 50 mg Niacin twice a day, OR I would take 2 heaping tablespoons Nutritional Yeast Flakes mixed into water, soup, broths, or other foods per day; Niacin is already in Nutritional Yeast Flakes.
Vitamin C	Wild Source Vitamin C capsules, along with selenium and hydrangea root from Dr. Clark's company	1,000 mg 3 times a day = 3,000 mg total; I started with small amounts and I slowly increased them to avoid loose stools
Vitamin E	Non-synthetic mixture (the letter "D" or "d" in front of the different types; aids the body in utilizing hydrogen peroixide	200 IU twice a day, or 400 IU once a day
Trace Minerals & Sodium plus Chloride	A "good" ocean sea salt, i.e. Celtic brand	1 teaspoon spread throughout the day

Niacin (B3) – I purchased a separate tablet of niacin (B3) because my Vitamin B Complex product contained niacinamide, which is a synthetic non-flushing form. "True" Niacin (B3) causes a flush, including itching and redness, which lasts up to an hour, but I learned this means it was helping me, and I learned it is nothing to be concerned about.

I learned to buy non-flushing niacin. Niacin is available in 50 mg, 100 mg, and 500 mg tablets so I learned to be careful which one I bought; it should be 50 mg, or cut 100 mg in half. Some people need to start with 25 mg or less and slowly increase it so their flush isn't so severe.

** Taken from http://healingnaturallybybee.com/articles/supp5.php

CHAPTER 42

Medicinal Herbal Teas: Keys to Long Life

Therefore whosoever hears these sayings of mine, and does them, I will liken him unto a wise man, which built his house upon a rock.—Matthew 7:24

According to Dr. Clark, medicinal teas will serve amazingly well in restoring health, as well as proving to be a protective barrier from future disease. There are a multitude of herbs beneficial to the body. I have listed the few I have become familiar with, but there are many more. Using the herbs listed below will prevent and help heal many infections, according to Dr. Clark. She claimed these infections can surface as the result of the toxic die-off of bacteria-producing germs and have the potential of slowing recovery time.

Dr. Clark advised you select a number of different ones, and drink them daily. She recommended the herbs be placed in the freezer for twenty-four hours before being used.

- Birch bark: 1 cup of tea twice a day or 1 capsule 2 times a day
- Boneset: 2 cups of tea a day or 1 capsule 3 times a day
- Burdock: 2 cups of tea a day or 1 capsule 3 times a day
- Chaga: 2 cups of the tea a day or 1 capsule 3 times a day
- Epazote: 2 cups of tea a day or 1 capsule 3 times a day
- Eucalyptus: 2 cups of tea a day or 1 capsule 3 times a day

- Larch: 2 cups of tea a day or 1 capsule 3 times a day
- Pau d'Arco: 2 cups of tea a day or 2 capsules 3 times a day
- Cayenne: take 1 capsule 2 times a day; inhibits tumor cell growth
- Juice of Wild Oreganol: pour 3 tablespoons into hot water and drink as a tea.

I learned from Dr. Clark's book, *The Cure & Prevention of all Cancers,* the advantage of drinking the teas while a person suffers with cancer is the teas are instrumental in helping to wash the cancer-causing germs quickly from the body.

She recommended making no less than 2.5 quarts of urine in twenty-four hours and no more than four quarts while washing out the cancer. The intake of fluids should be half the body weight in ounces. For instance, if you weigh 120 pounds, your fluid intake should be no less than 60 ounces a day. I learned it was important for me to stay hydrated, but I did not force myself to drink large amounts of water. I found Pau d'Arco is an awesome herb in the fight against cancer as it is an antifungal.

There have been times I have experienced underlying itching in my breast as the result of what I had been eating. I immediately "cleaned up my diet" and began to take Pau d'Arco, 3 capsules every few hours, along with the Juice of Wild Oreganol. All of the symptoms quickly went away. This is an extremely powerful herb in the fight against cancer. After I treated with 35% H202, which I have written about in Chapter 22, I no longer suffered with any cancer symptoms and no longer needed to use any type of remedy, regardless of what I ate.

Essiac tea, also known as Flor Essence, is a remarkable product which has been used by many to be healed of cancer. Essiac contains a blend of some of the teas mentioned at the beginning of this chapter. It is an ancient herbal remedy which was brought to light by a Canadian nurse named Rene Caisse. Essiac is Caisse spelled backwards. This tea is available in many health food stores. The tea can be brewed and drank or it can be taken in a convenient capsule form.

Essiac is an herbal remedy comprised of sheep sorrel, sometimes called sour grass; burdock root; slippery elm bark; rhubarb root; and other potent herbs, such as watercress, blessed thistle, red clover, and kelp. It can be taken safely over long periods of time in the case of illness or as a tonic to insure good health. There are no ill side effects, and it can be taken along with any other therapies.

There is an available book entitled Essiac Report. Within the book are certified documents and statements from prominent doctors who have endorsed its use. Reports are given as to what medical institutions have tested Essiac and the results. It contains documented case histories of terminal patients who claim to have been completely healed of cancer by using Essiac. It also provides information on how it can be used as a method of cancer prevention. I have a friend who takes two capsules of Essiac every day as a preventative measure.

CHAPTER 43

The Natural Solution for the Human Papilloma Virus

For You, O God, have girded me with strength unto
the battle; and You, O God, have subdued under
me those that rose up against me.—Psalm 18:39

The human papilloma virus, HPV, a wart virus, is the most common sexually transmitted infectious disease. HPV is considered a serious health crisis, as conventional medicine offers no lasting or effective cure.

Although contracting the wart virus is commonly associated with sexual contact, that is by no means the only way one may become infected. According to the American Family Physician, a periodical, many people have reported to their doctor their small children were also infected by the virus simply by normal family contact.

The periodical states HPV can be contracted from such sources as soiled bedding and towels, worn clothing, public saunas, tanning beds and by contact with a wart on an infected individual, whenever the bare skin is exposed to the virus. All it takes is a weakened immune system. When a person already suffers with cancer, the likelihood of their contracting a virus of any kind greatly increases.

The inexpensive solution I learned about, which will effectively treat all strains of this virus, is 35% food grade hydrogen peroxide. I detailed my experience with hydrogen peroxide in Chapter 22.

HPV has become so widespread that it has taken on epidemic proportions. It is associated with a number of serious health issues, including many types of cancer.

I learned from reading *The Cure & Prevention of all Cancers* that this virus attaches itself to the cancer-causing germ in order to enter the body. The cancer-causing germ serves as a catalyst or facilitator for the virus to move about. When the cancer-causing germ is eliminated, the virus is left without a means to be transported throughout the body, thus weakening the virus and its outbreak.

The Alotek Company sells a product called beta mannan; this product is about $40 per bottle, and the company recommends you take 3 bottles the first month. When properly taken, beta mannan will boost the body's immune system, and the body's own immune system will subdue the virus. If beta mannan is taken in conjunction with the herbal germ cleanse in Chapter 19 results will be noticed in a matter of just a few hours.

If a person who is suffering with cancer contracts HPV, beta mannan will not be effective in subduing the virus.

Using 35% food grade hydrogen peroxide and adding 3 to 5 drops of black walnut tincture to the first couple of doses is far less expensive than using beta mannan and is so effective that it will allow even a person with cancer to subdue the virus, as H202 boosts the immune system. The use of 35% food grade hydrogen peroxide, H202, boosts the immune system enough to allow the body to completely heal. The method of treating with H202 is contained in Chapter 22. It is important to remember that although the immune system has subdued the virus, and there are no longer any visible symptoms of its presence, the virus might still be carried in the body.

There are now at least 100 strains of the human papilloma virus, which have been identified. Some of the strains of the wart virus cause warts to grow inside and outside the genitalia and the rectum; other strains of the virus result in warts in other areas of the body, sometimes in the mouth or throat and often on the hands and feet. The strains of HPV, which present the highest risk for a woman's cervical health and are associated with the development of precancerous cells, referred to as dysplasia, in the cervix are 16, 18, 31 and 45.

As well as being linked to the condition of cervical cancer, HPV is also found to be the culprit in the development of cancer of the vulva, vagina, penis, rectum, oropharynx (the back of the throat, including the base of the tongue and the tonsils.) In rare cases, the virus can result in recurrent respiratory papillomatosis, RRP, warts in the throat, resulting in the voice becoming chronically hoarse.

In my research, I learned that besides the telltale signs of the unsightly warts which can potentially completely cover the genitalia, as well as grow deep inside the body, HPV is also known to cause painful stinging sensations throughout the body, along with severe itching in the rectum, the initial symptom which most often prompts the first visit to a physician.

In addition to the link between HPV and the development of a number of cancers, researchers have now concluded there is a direct connection between periodontal disease and the human papilloma virus. Researchers estimate that as much as 79% of the populace who were infected with HPV also developed periodontal disease. I learned treating with 35% food grade hydrogen peroxide will also heal the periodontal disease associated with this virus.

According to the medical periodical I read, it is possible to have the virus and be totally unaware of its presence, as the warts may grow deep inside the vagina, within the bladder, as well as the urethra of the penis, out of sight of the sufferer. Because of its widespread presence, it is now a standard practice for an ob/gyn to order a test for the presence of HPV when their patients visit for a checkup.

I learned from Dr. Clark's book, *The Cure & Prevention of all Cancers,* that eating dairy products can trigger an HPV outbreak.

CHAPTER 44

The Natural Solution for the Herpes Virus

The angel of the Lord encamps round about them
that fear Him and delivers them.—Psalm 34:7

I learned treating with 35% food grade hydrogen peroxide, H202, would also eliminate the herpes virus, and that it was extremely important to follow through with the entire course of H202, as outlined in Chapter 22.

Below is what I learned from reading the writings of Dr. Hulda Clark. Included in the herpes virus category are a variety of strains: Herpes Simplex Virus (HSV) 1 & 2, Epstein-Barr virus (EBV), shingles or Chicken Pox (Varicella zoster, Cytomegalovirus (CMV), as well as a growing list of newly discovered strains of the virus.

According to Dr. Clark, herpes simplex virus 1 is the virus that breaks out around or inside the mouth. It is commonly referred to as a cold sore because it often appears following a cold. A cold sore is an indication of a weakened immune system.

Herpes simplex virus 2 breaks out in the genital area. It is often blamed on promiscuous sex. Dr. Clark claimed that though it indeed is sexually transmitted, the virus itself enters the body by piggy-backing or riding on cancer-causing germs which are exchanged during sexual relations. What this translates to, according to Dr. Clark, is that if the germs are eliminated, the virus is limited in its ability to attack the body. Chapter

271

19 outlines Dr. Clark's recommended method of eliminating the cancer-causing germ.

I shared this information with a gentleman who was experiencing an outbreak of shingles, and he told me that using the herbal germ cleanse had been extremely effective in quickly clearing up the shingles outbreak.

Herpes lives in the nerve centers (ganglia), and it is from the nerve centers that the body is attacked by the virus after the initial infection. Dr. Clark claimed a strong immune system can destroy them as quickly as they emerge. However a meal which includes moldy foods or aflatoxins will overwhelm the white blood cells and result in a herpes outbreak. Dr. Clark recommended the detox trio, vitamin C, selenium and germanium to combat this problem.

Dr. Clark asserted that just eating a bruised apple could trigger a herpes outbreak. She found that when the virus is triggered, it is allowed to multiply and travel along the nerve fiber to the skin. Triggers are things that put the nerve centers to work, such as: Sudden cold and heat, trauma from chafing and friction. In order to reduce the Herpes 1 outbreaks, Dr. Clark recommends avoiding beverages which contain ice cubes; to avoid eating hot soup with a metal spoon; as well as avoiding tweezing hairs near the mouth.

In the case of Herpes 2 she said to avoid wearing tight synthetic underwear.

Dr. Clark recommended you begin your prevention program by raising the immunity of your skin. This means not using products with toxins on your skin, i.e., soaps, perfumes, lotions, et cetera. She suggested the use of only pure and natural products. The Miracle II products are an excellent choice.

You can locate an almost endless amount of information on the Internet with regard to directions on how to concoct your own homemade shampoo, body creams, mascara, and more. Just simply using organic extra virgin coconut oil as a skin cleanser and skin softener is a great beginning. Do laundry with borax and washing soda, eliminating commercial laundry detergent as a toxic source, which Dr. Clark claims can prompt a herpes outbreak.

She advises that as soon as you feel that warning of a tingling sensation, regardless of the type of herpes outbreak, take action. Chapters 18 and

19, which include the detox trio and the herbal germ cleanse, is what Dr. Clark recommended. She also recommended that you immediately take a cayenne capsule and 8 L-lysine tablets (500 mg. each). Treating with 35% Food Grade Hydrogen Peroxide will prevent herpes outbreaks. All products mentioned in this chapter can be purchased online from www.ibeatcancers.com.

According to Dr. Clark, the cayenne slows down the travel of the virus along the nerve, allowing the L-lysine time to have full impact on the affronting virus.

The Alotek Company, which produces the beta mannan product, claims that many people who suffer with the herpes virus are helped by taking beta mannan.

I read that bathing in a warm bath which contains a quart of 3% food grade hydrogen peroxide will quickly ease the pain of a shingles outbreak. The article advises adding an additional quart of 3% food grade hydrogen peroxide once the bath cools and adding more hot water to a comfortable temperature.

CHAPTER 45

Useful Tools in Waging War against Disease

And Moses spoke to the people, saying, arm
yourselves for the war.—Numbers 31:3

I learned that there are numerous pieces of very effective equipment available to help you wage war against cancer or just plain remain healthy. None of these products diagnose a disease; that is the role of your physician.

The following list contains a small selection of some of the quality equipment you can purchase by going to my website, www.ibeatcancers.com, where you will find a link to these items.

- A selection of far infrared pads and cushions: These far infrared products utilize a unique technology which expands capillaries, assisting in increased blood flow and circulation; this means these wonderful items will aid in quickly reducing and even eliminating pain and promote healing. They can be packed easily for travel, allowing you to get a good night's sleep on a strange bed. The soft far infrared pads, which are equipped with a built-in timer, aid in relaxing the body and help you to get a better night's sleep. I found these items helped me quickly get out of discomfort and throbbing pain and into a relaxed condition, eliminating any need for over-the-counter pain killers or sleeping aids!

- A lymphatic cleansing machine: Developed by a renowned Chinese medical visionary, this unique device massages the internal organs and all body systems. Fifteen minutes on this machine is equivalent to 10,000 steps in terms of body oxygenation. Oxygenation aids in prevention of disease and boosts the capacity of bone marrow to produce red blood cells. Because of its ability to help cleanse the lymphatic system, it aids in expediting wound healing.

- A far infrared sauna hothouse: This portable piece of equipment allows you to place the far infrared directly over any area of the body experiencing pain and in need of healing. It elevates body temperature, which stimulates blood circulation, accelerating the metabolic exchange between the body and blood vessels to relieve pain and is wonderfully effective in speeding the healing process. This is an awesome device to speed healing after surgery, as well as accelerating the healing of infected cuts, abrasions and broken bones. A far infrared sauna reportedly aids in ridding the body of dangerous toxins. The hothouse is convenient to use, either on the floor or bed and can be used in conjunction with the far infrared pad to intensify its efficiency. Simply drape a blanket over the top of the hothouse, which traps in the heat. I sustained a cut on my finger, which was so damaged it could not be stitched together. I used the hothouse, together with the far infrared pad, and my finger was healed in just a few days. Everyone who saw the wound, including a nurse friend of mine, was amazed by how quickly it healed, leaving no scar.

- An electrical frequency device: I have found the ERE to be an awesome device. This device helps reconnect broken or damaged electrical circuits within the body by stimulating it with the correct waveform, current and frequency. When there is pain in the body, there is electrical resistance, meaning the electrical signals between cells are suppressed. Consistent use of this machine can help restore the flow of electricity through the painful areas of the body and allow the body to be pain free. This device comes with electrodes, which can be placed on painful areas of the body, but should not be placed directly over the heart. I found that use of this device helped prevent chronic sciatic pain. Relieves pain associated with neuropathy and arthritis. This device helps to relieve carpal tunnel syndrome and muscle spasms. Expedites healing of bruises. Promotes the breakdown of fat cells and aids in detoxification.

- An electrical energy belt: The electric potential in the human body reduces with age, and the reduction of electric potential can trigger illness. For this reason, it is necessary to increase the electrical potential to improve your health by building the immune system and insure maximum longevity.

- A device to improve eyesight: This specially formulated device called Power Eyes combines air pressure, heat compression, and vibrating massage, which can benefit blood circulation around the eye area. This is also good for the metabolic process around the eyes and helps eliminate dark circles and fine lines. Power Eyes promote a good night's sleep.

- A unique sauna bed: The ultimate total health spa experience built into a specially designed massage table. A safe, simple and a natural way to achieve good health!

Epilogue

Jesus Is the Answer to Every Need

The Lord thy God in the midst of thee is
mighty; He will save, He will rejoice over thee
with joy; He will rest in His love, He will joy over
thee with singing.—Zephaniah 3:17 KJV

As many as accepted Jesus as Lord, to them
gave He the power to become the sons and
daughters of God.—John 1:12 KJV

Making the decision to invite Jesus to be your Savior brings you into fellowship with a gracious, forgiving, merciful, and loving God. God does not consider us guilty for our wrongdoings in any way when we accept His son, as Jesus took the punishment for the sins of all people throughout all generations. The scripture states that whosoever calls upon the name of the Lord Jesus shall be saved from destruction.

When you ask Jesus to be the Lord of your life and you earnestly follow Him with all of your heart, He causes you to prosper in every facet of your life; as you walk in His path, He surrounds you with His favor and blessings.

Jesus has called and lovingly beckoned to all of humankind by saying, "Come unto me all you who are weary and heavy laden, and I will give you rest" (Matthew 11:28 KJV).

Saint Paul wrote in a letter to the Romans, "If you shall confess with your mouth the Lord Jesus, and shall believe in your heart, that God has raised him from the dead, you shall be *saved*" (Romans 10:9).

I want you to know God gave me no rest until I completed this book. His desire for you is to live and not die, to enable you to declare He is the God that hears and cares and has made every provision for healing because of His great love.

God wants the best for His people—to make them leaders in life, rather than mindless followers. God wants to bless your life and fill it with good things. He longs to make you whole—body, mind, and spirit.

The sin of Adam and Eve in the Garden of Eden created a gap between God and humankind, and the Bible clearly tells us Jesus is the ONLY WAY possible to bridge or close this gap.

I recall as a young woman hearing the word *saved*. I thought to myself, *saved*? What does that mean? *Saved* from what? In my small circle of life, all of the people I knew who claimed to be *saved* appeared to live a defeated life. The outward appearance of their lives did not at all entice me to follow their example. I did not understand the things of God.

Despite these misgivings, at 31 years of age, I accompanied my newly *saved* parents to a different kind of church from the one in which I had been raised. I heard the Gospel preached for the very first time. Although I did not fully understand the entire concept of Christianity at the time, I was so strongly drawn to it that I was just like a fish being caught up into a giant net. Something supernatural happened to me that day. I began weeping uncontrollably and embraced the love of God. Oh, how sweet is that memory. What a wonderful presence of peace that covered me.

I gradually began learning what *saved* actually means. God loves people. God *saves* people from anything that would hinder or destroy them! He wants us to live without any shackles, bondages, addictions or destructive habits which would prevent us from being all He created us to be! He is powerful! He is able to do all things! He delights in us!

God wants to protect us from anything and everything that would defeat or destroy us. He desires that we excel in every aspect of our lives. His desire is for us to live in joy and victory! He answers when we cry to Him, asking for His divine intervention! His desire for us is that we suffer no lack; that we have everything we need.

The Bible tells us that God wants us to prosper to the point of excess, not so we can hoard earthly possessions, but to be able to give into His kingdom, to help the poor, to remove the pain and suffering of others. He wants us to reveal His love to others!

Our great God does not steal from us, kill us, nor destroy us, but it is His enemy and our enemy, Satan and his minions, who conspire against us. Many people unintentionally discredit God when they blame Him for their losses. God wants to increase us more and more. He is not a thief.

Remember reading my dream about breast cancer, where the demons were carrying me and the little girls away? Well, God was the one who stopped them! He *saved* me! He is an awesome God! He is a faithful father to all of His children!

I am asking you to make a decision today. I am asking you to pray this simple prayer with me. I am asking you to invite this wonderful God I have described to become involved in your life so He can *save* you.

PRAYER

Dear Lord Jesus, please forgive me for the sins I have committed. I thank you, Lord, for giving your life in exchange for mine when you died on the cross for my sins. You did this because of Your great love for me and Your desire to set me free from anything that would prevent me from living a joyful life. I thank you that as I pray this prayer, the sinless blood you shed on a cruel cross washes me clean from sin and breaks down the strongholds of unbelief and rebellion which have been part of my very own carnal nature.

Thank you for your forgiveness and thank you for giving me a new heart so I may come to know you, as you patiently teach me to walk in your ways. Thank you for restoring my health and opening unto me your beautiful kingdom of heaven. I accept you as my *Savior*, Jesus, the one who has reconciled me to a holy God. I thank you for *saving* me; that you lovingly and willingly have done for me what I am incapable of doing for myself. I ask that you fill me with Your Holy Spirit and teach me to hear your voice. Lord, I want to fulfill all you have planned for my life. Amen.

If you prayed that prayer, you are now a new person in Christ Jesus. Old things have passed away, and all things are made new again. You now have a brand new beginning in your life. Get to know your heavenly Father by reading the book He has provided for His people, the Bible. Get yourself a Bible that is easy to read. Yes, men wrote it, but they are writings inspired by God's Holy Spirit. I recommend The Living Bible translation. Begin to read the books of the Gospel, a word that literally means "good news"—Matthew, Mark, Luke, and John.

Find yourself a Bible believing church to attend. If things don't feel right at the first one you attend, keep trying until you find the right fit. The right church should be warm, friendly, fun, with wonderful praise and worship and Bible-based teachings that enable you to grow! Your new church should believe in all of the gifts of the Holy Spirit, such as healing and prophecy.

Be sure to send me your own healing testimony so it can be used to encourage others. Contact me at www.ibeatcancers.com. I care very deeply about you and want to hear your story of restored health as well as your decision to follow our wonderful *Savior*, Jesus.

About the Author

Mary Rock is a woman who passionately loves God. She has been called a thoroughbred intercessor, having experienced some phenomenal answers to prayer in her 30-plus years as a Christian. As a speaker, Mary brings a fresh message with power and candor. Her disarming sense of humor brings laughter and freedom, as she shares her many, many trials and the eventual triumphs, which manifested due to the faithfulness of God. Mary's deepest desire is to inspire others to take up the authority given to them by Jesus Christ, to walk in the freedom and liberty He has provided. As a teacher, she has remarkable insight into the Word of God and its practical application to everyday life. She walks in a prophetic anointing and has been used by God in winning the lost and ministering to those who are bound by spirits of addiction and infirmity.

Above all, Mary Rock ministers to the body of Christ in love, with comfort and encouragement.

Mary is a minister licensed by The Covenant Center in Lakeland, Florida, pastored by Richard & Becky Maisenbacher. She is available for speaking and teaching engagements. Contact Mary at www.ibeatcancers.com

Index

Printed in the United States
By Bookmasters